ANTI-INFLAMMATORY DIET IN 21

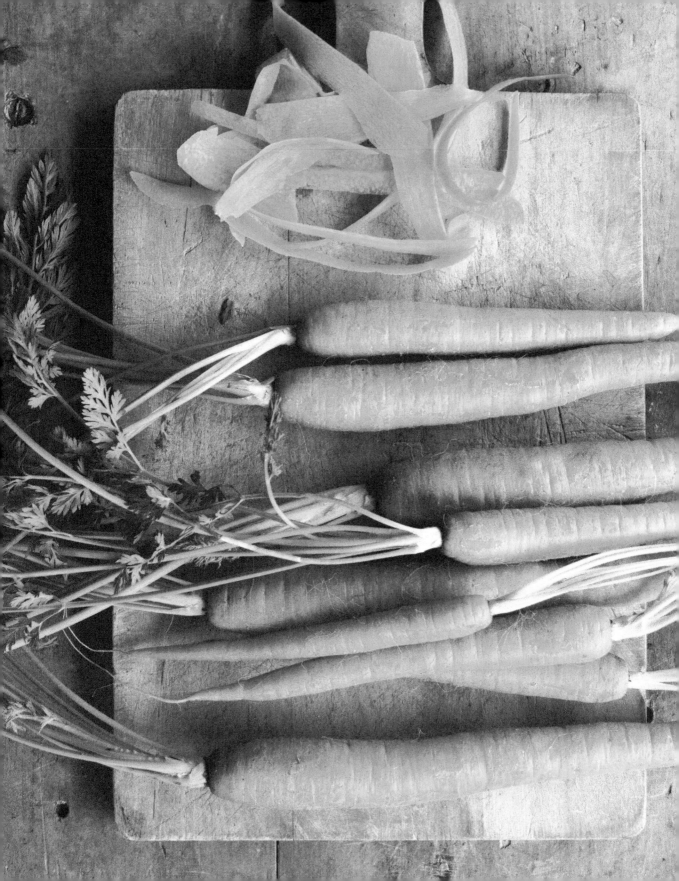

ANTI-INFLAMMATORY DIET in 21

100 Recipes, 5 Ingredients, and 3 Weeks to Fight Inflammation

SONDI BRUNER

ROCKRIDGE
PRESS

For general information on our other products and services or to obtain technical support, please contact our Customer Care Department within the U.S. at (866) 744-2665, or outside the U.S. at (510) 253-0500.

Rockridge Press publishes its books in a variety of electronic and print formats. Some content that appears in print may not be available in electronic books, and vice versa.

TRADEMARKS: Rockridge Press and the Rockridge Press logo are trademarks or registered trademarks of Callisto Media, Inc., and/or its affiliates, in the United States and other countries, and may not be used without written permission. All other trademarks are the property of their respective owners. Rockridge Press is not associated with any product or vendor mentioned in this book.

Cover photographs © (front) StockFood/ Amanda Stockley; (back, top to bottom) StockFood/Jean-Christophe Riou; StockFood/ George Crudo; Stocksy/Nataša Mandić

Interior photographs © Stocksy/Sara Remington, p. 2; Stocksy/Roel David Smart, p. 6; Stocksy/Jeff Wasserman, p. 10; Stocksy/ Alberto Bogo, p. 28; Stockfood/Gräfe & Unzer Verlag/Jörn Rynio, p. 50; Stockfood/ Lars Ranek, p. 57; Stocksy/Pavel Gramatikov, p. 66; Stocksy/Ina Peters, p. 73; Stocksy/ Marta Muñoz-Calero Calderon, p .82; Stocksy/ Nataša Mandić, p. 91; Stockfood/Winfried Heinze, p. 100; StockFood/Jalag/Janne Peters, p. 110; StockFood/George Crudo, p. 120; Stocksy/David Illini, p. 130; StockFood/ Sporrer/Skowronek, p. 149; StockFood/Jean-Christophe Riou, p. 162; Stocksy/Ruth Black, p.169; StockFood/Jo Kirchherr, p.174; Stocksy/Canan Czemmel, p. 186

ISBN: Print 978-1-62315-673-2
eBook 978-1-62315-674-9

CONTENTS

*To those dealing with a chronic, inflammatory condition:
I understand. I empathize. I know. It can be mentally and
physically exhausting, not to mention excruciatingly
painful. The good news? The food on your plate is powerful.
Choose well. Choose wisely. Choose health.*

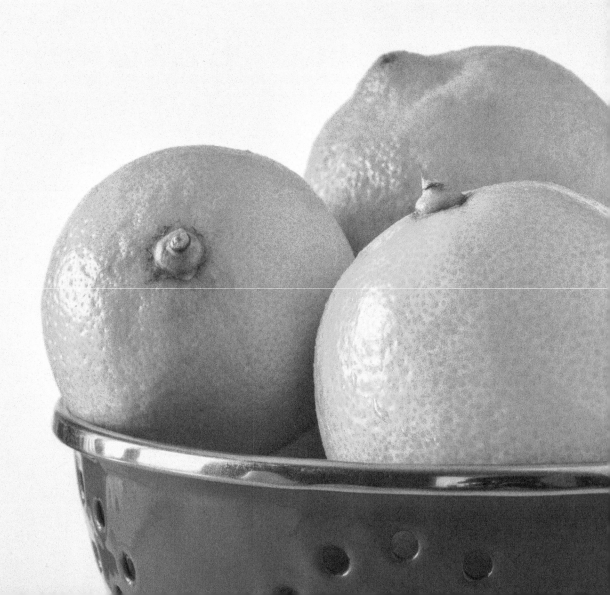

THE ANTI-INFLAMMATORY PATH TO GOOD HEALTH

EAT VEGETABLES AND FRUITS. Virtually every fruit and vegetable on the planet is an anti-inflammatory all-star that contains a wide range of nutrients that support health—including antioxidants, fiber, vitamins, minerals, and protein.

CONSUME HEALTHY FATS, PARTICULARLY OMEGA-3S. Fat is not to be feared—it's definitely your friend in the fight against inflammation. Focus on a specific type of fat called omega-3 fatty acids, as these are especially anti-inflammatory and available in food sources such as flaxseed, walnuts, hemp seeds, salmon, chia seeds, and even vegetables (particularly the dark green leafy ones).

EAT PLENTY OF PROTEIN. Protein, which is built from amino acids, is an important nutrient in an anti-inflammatory diet for a variety of reasons. Amino acids are essential for growth, healing, and repair of tissues, plus they produce hormones, the antibodies that battle inflammation, and the enzymes that help digestion.

MANAGE STRESS. It's tough for your body to heal inflammation when you're under stress. Research has proven that chronic stress prevents our bodies from regulating inflammation properly, which can lead to many diseases.

SLEEP SEVEN TO EIGHT HOURS PER NIGHT. Lack of sleep is associated with higher levels of inflammation. Quality sleep is important. It's the time when we imprint what we've learned throughout the day, and essential to repair, recharge, and regenerate body tissues.

INTRODUCTION

TO BE BLUNT, INFLAMMATION IS NO PICNIC,
BUT YOU PROBABLY ALREADY KNOW THAT.

Body parts hurt. Energy levels are low. Your brain feels like it's struggling through wet cement. There are embarrassing bumps and blemishes on your skin where they shouldn't be. And, as if the physical symptoms weren't enough, to fix the problem you've been told to eliminate foods you love.

I've been there.

My eighteen-year-old self thought I was invincible. Even after being diagnosed with Crohn's disease I didn't change a single thing about my diet or lifestyle. I continued to consume bread, fluffy bagels, white rice, cheese, muffins, cookies, ice cream, candy, and chocolate without a thought. Did you notice there are no vegetables on this list? I scoffed at them.

I didn't realize it at the time, but this steady diet of sugar and processed foods only worsened my inflammatory symptoms. As the years went by, my medications grew stronger and I got sicker, bouncing in and out of emergency rooms with bowel obstructions. At twenty-three, I underwent surgery to remove a foot of small bowel. And after all this—would you believe I *still* wasn't propelled to change my diet or lifestyle?

I reached a point in my mid-twenties where I virtually had stopped eating to control the awful symptoms—raging diarrhea, perpetual swelling with painful bloating—I could barely keep my eyes open. When my gastroenterologist declared, "Well, you look fine," I promptly hurried to a naturopathic doctor for a second opinion. She, finally, completely changed my diet and I, finally, began to feel better and understand the power of food.

An anti-inflammatory diet has been a life changer for me—and the elimination of gluten and dairy has been especially transformative. I'm able to manage and control my symptoms by what I choose to eat, and have experienced tremendous improvements in my quality of life.

Be forewarned: it isn't easy at first. When I began this journey, my naturopath prescribed a strict elimination diet that excluded wheat, dairy, sugar, alcohol, fruit, yeast, and all processed foods.

As someone who didn't know how to cook and who ate everything from a box, can, or sealed plastic bag, following this diet was radical, overwhelming, and *hard*.

It was also the best thing I ever did. As time went by I noticed not only a reduction in symptoms, but I also learned valuable cooking skills that helped me prepare healthy, nourishing foods from scratch. This cleared the path to better health, and set the stage for the work I'm doing today. Ten years ago, I had no idea that I would leave my career, write a food blog, start my own business, and help clients develop the tools they need to facilitate their wellness. You just never know where your choices may lead you.

Holding this book in your hands brings you one step closer to improving your health and reducing inflammation. Congratulations. Each subsequent choice you make after today will lead you down your own path to wellness. Some days, it might seem like you're moving inch by inch, and on others you'll feel as if you're leaping for miles; but one thing I know for certain is that you can make it happen; just keep moving forward.

In these pages you'll find tools to help reduce inflammation and support your immune system, including menu plans, detailed food lists, cooking tips, and 100 easy-to-make recipes using just five primary ingredients. These recipes contain limited ingredients so meals will be convenient, quick, and easy, while simultaneously supporting your health goals. In case you're worried, the recipes don't compromise on flavor—there is a wide variety of tastes to enjoy, too. You won't miss your old diet in the least because you'll be too busy reveling in the abundance of delicious food choices you have.

Good health lies in your hands. Embrace it and be proud of the steps you're taking to improve your life.

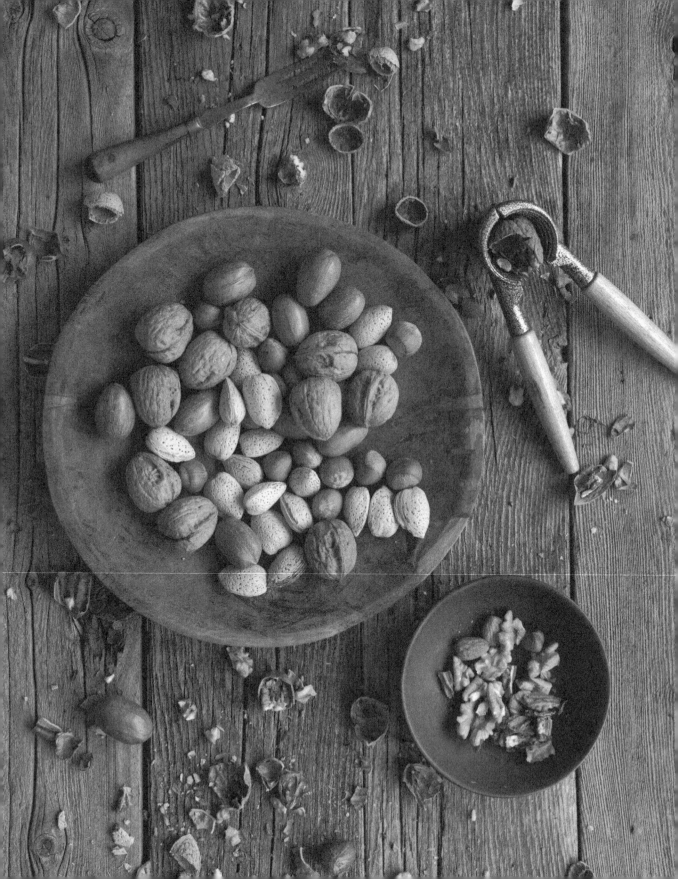

SOOTHING CHRONIC INFLAMMATION 1

If you've ever had a cold, a cut on your finger, a rash, or a bruise, then you've experienced inflammation. In urgent situations, inflammation is incredibly useful—similar to emergency personnel being dispatched to an accident. However, if inflammation becomes chronic or our immune system fails to work properly, people can develop a host of diseases that can impact day-to-day existence, including family lives, social lives, and careers.

However, with education and information you can take control of your health and prevent or manage your inflammation.

One of the best ways to reduce inflammation is by eating a healthy, anti-inflammatory diet. Nature is filled with foods that contain potent, inflammation-fighting nutrients. When you fill your plate with this soothing fare, you'll begin to calm the angry symptoms that plague you.

THE ROOT OF MANY HEALTH PROBLEMS

Inflammation is a growing problem worldwide for a variety of reasons, including poor nutrition, toxins in the environment, genetics, widespread medication use, stress, and limited physical activity.

The immune system is intricately involved in the inflammatory process, sending chemical messengers to fix the damage when it occurs. For example, if you cut your finger your immune system swings into action and sends out chemical messengers to destroy bacteria and initiate the healing process.

Acute inflammation is short lived, and essential to survival. *Chronic inflammation* occurs when we are unable to defeat the original injury, the irritant continues to be present in the body, or, as is the case with autoimmune diseases, the body begins to attack healthy tissue.

Inflammation is at the root of many diseases and conditions. Health problems linked to inflammation include:

INFLAMMATORY BOWEL DISEASE (IBD). This includes Crohn's disease and colitis, which occur when the digestive tract becomes inflamed, leading to poor digestion and absorption of nutrients.

HEART DISEASE. An umbrella term for numerous conditions that impact the cardiovascular system. Many common heart issues involve damage to the arteries and blood vessels, which can lead to inflammation and reduced blood flow.

OBESITY. Excess weight can cause a range of inflammatory conditions, including osteoarthritis, heart disease, diabetes, cancer, high blood pressure, and gallstones.

RHEUMATOID ARTHRITIS AND OSTEOARTHRITIS. Rheumatoid arthritis occurs when the body attacks its own tissues, causing inflammation in the joints. Osteoarthritis also involves inflammation, but its cause is wear and tear in the joints over time.

ALLERGIES. Food, drugs, animals, plants, mold, latex, or other toxins can cause the immune system to overreact, leading to a host of uncomfortable symptoms.

ASTHMA. This inflammatory disease of the lungs involves coughing, shortness of breath, and chest tightness.

LUPUS. This autoimmune disease involves the body attacking its own tissues, leading to inflammation in many different parts of the body.

HASHIMOTO'S DISEASE. This is an autoimmune disease in which the immune system attacks and damages the thyroid, which can lead to swelling of the thyroid (called a goiter), weight gain, fatigue, dry skin, and depression.

DIABETES. This occurs when the body doesn't produce enough insulin, or can't effectively use the insulin it creates. Complications from diabetes involve inflammation, such as obesity, atherosclerosis, and foot ulcers.

CANCER. This disease happens when abnormal cells grow, invade different parts of the body, and hijack healthy cells. Once the immune system is activated, inflammation can become widespread. It also works the other way; chronic inflammation can leave the immune system and the body susceptible to cancerous changes.

CELIAC DISEASE. Having this autoimmune disease means the body can't process gluten, leading to damage in the small intestine. Untreated celiac disease can lead to other inflammatory conditions like diabetes and dermatitis herpetiformis, an uncomfortable skin condition.

MULTIPLE SCLEROSIS (MS). This autoimmune disease of the nervous system results in the protective coatings on nerve cells—called myelin sheaths—being attacked and damaged. This can cause vision problems, disrupted motor function, dizziness, and muscle weakness.

SKIN DISEASES. Inflammatory skin conditions such as eczema, acne, rosacea, and psoriasis can lead to redness, itchiness, dry skin, skin bumps, and pimples.

HEADACHES. Tension headaches usually involve a steady, dull pain or pressure, while migraines tend to have a throbbing or pounding quality.

BRAIN DISORDERS. Neurologist Dr. David Perlmutter, author of *Grain Brain*, links inflammation and the consumption of sugar and carbs to a variety of brain disorders including dementia, ADHD, anxiety, depression, and epilepsy.

FIGHTING INFLAMMATION WITH SMART DIETARY CHOICES

Keep Your Eyes on the Prize

We all make bad choices occasionally, but we learn from them and grow. Forgive yourself for those bad food choices in the past and start fresh— literally! Following an anti-inflammatory diet means moving forward. Guilt or regret will not help and will only hold you in place—and induce stress, which we know is not conducive to reducing inflammation. Focus on the good—no, great—things ahead.

Some health benefits you will reap after adopting an anti-inflammatory diet include:

REDUCTION IN SYMPTOMS. As you consistently choose to fill your plate with soothing, anti-inflammatory food, you'll likely notice your symptoms diminish. If your symptoms are especially cumbersome and intrusive, this will be a great relief!

MORE ENERGY. When you fuel your body with the variety of macro- and micronutrients it needs, you'll feel more energized and ready to tackle daily activities.

IMPROVED DIGESTION. Good health begins with good digestion. Since the recipes in this book all have minimal ingredients, the result is less work for your body to process them. You may notice fewer digestive problems, such as acid reflux, bloating, cramping, or gas, while on an anti-inflammatory diet. Also, 70 percent of the immune system is located in and around the digestive tract. A healthy digestive tract means a healthy immune system, too!

INCREASED FOCUS. You may feel more clear-headed, more attentive, and sharper—always a good thing.

FEWER ACHES AND PAINS. Our immune response naturally produces redness, swelling, or pain so the chemical messengers can sweep away the injury and heal the body. An anti-inflammatory diet can lead to fewer aches and pains, as that redness or swelling won't happen in the first place.

A STRENGTHENED IMMUNE SYSTEM. Widespread inflammation means your body is on high alert, sending out inflammatory messengers on a regular basis. Without the constant fire of inflammation to douse, your immune system will work more efficiently.

FOODS THAT WORSEN THE IMMUNE SYSTEM

Food plays a key role in the inflammatory response. Our food choices can soothe, or worsen, inflammation. First, let's look at *foods to avoid* on an anti-inflammatory diet, as well as unexpected or hidden sources for these inflammation-inducing foods.

Gluten

Gluten is a protein found in wheat, wheat germ, barley, rye, spelt, kamut, farro, bulgur, semolina, farina, and triticale. People with celiac disease mount an immune response to a specific protein in gluten called *gliadin*. As a result, the immune cells destroy the microvilli in the small intestine, which are responsible for absorbing nutrients.

For people without celiac, gluten can still be incredibly hard to process, and can aggravate most inflammatory conditions. Some effects of consuming gluten include digestive upset, brain fog, sinus problems, joint pain, blood sugar imbalances, hormonal imbalances, and skin conditions.

Dairy

Most people don't produce the lactase enzyme required to digest the lactose sugars in cow's milk, leading to bloating, gas, and diarrhea.

Milk is a mucus-forming food and, when that mucus coats the digestive tract, it prevents nutrients from being absorbed. Dairy cows raised for conventional milk products are fed growth hormones and antibiotics, which can interfere with a person's hormonal balance and/or lead to inflammation. Finally, conventional dairy products are often loaded with sugar and preservatives (especially the low-fat ones) and this can further contribute to the inflammatory processes.

Corn

Corn is a common allergen, and it is also often genetically modified—about 90 percent of corn in the United States is genetically engineered, according to the GMO Compass website. Genetically modified organisms, or GMOs, are relatively new to our food system and can potentially pose serious risks to health. For example, they can suppress the immune system and encourage inflammation. Corn is ubiquitous in processed foods, as well—so if you're eating those foods, you're eating corn.

Soy

Similar to corn, this controversial bean is a common allergen, and GMO Compass reports that 93 percent of soy grown in the United States is genetically modified. In addition to the genetic modification, soy is high in *goitrogens*, compounds that can suppress thyroid function. Soy also contains antinutrients, such as *phytates* and *oxalates*, which interfere with our digestion and disrupt the endocrine system.

Peanuts

Another common allergen, peanuts contain a carcinogenic mold called *aflatoxin*, which can affect those with liver conditions or candida. Peanut crops are heavily treated with pesticides and this can lead to further inflammation or allergic reactions. They are also high in omega-6 fatty acids, a pro-inflammatory fat, and conventional peanut butters are often loaded with added sugar and trans fats.

Caffeine

Coffee propels the stomach to release its contents prematurely, injecting undigested food into the small intestine where it can aggravate the digestive tract. Caffeine can send blood sugar soaring, raise blood pressure and heart rate, suppress appetite, and disrupt sleep. Coffee also stresses the nervous system, which can interfere with the production of the anti-inflammatory hormone cortisol.

Alcohol

While the occasional glass of wine offers a hit of antioxidants, overall, excess alcohol consumption can increase the production of C-reactive protein (CRP), a marker of inflammation in the blood.

Many alcoholic beverages are chock-full of sugar, which can wreak havoc on our blood sugar levels, cause headaches, and suppress the immune system. Alcohol also destroys gut flora, an integral part of the digestive system. Poor intestinal flora can lead to a leaky gut, where particles of food break through the intestinal barrier and activate the immune system, inducing further inflammation and allergies.

Citrus Foods

Most citrus foods are acidic and can provoke inflammation in people with a variety of conditions such as gastroesophageal reflux disease (GERD), arthritis, and citrus sensitivities. To buffer their acidity in the body, we pull from our body's pool of soothing alkaline minerals such as calcium, magnesium, and potassium. An acidic environment can place undue stress on the body, leaving a person susceptible to disease.

However, lemons or limes can be a handy addition to an anti-inflammatory diet. They kick-start digestion, enhance liver detoxification, and once metabolized by the body, they leave alkaline minerals behind. Overall, though, avoid citrus.

Feedlot Animal Products

Conventional animal products induce inflammation for a variety of reasons. Animals are fed hormones and antibiotics. This not only contributes to inflammation but also to the growing worldwide problem of antibiotic resistance.

Feedlot animals are often fed fare that is different from their natural diet—mostly grains like wheat, GMO corn, and GMO soy. We know these are inflammatory. Grain-fed animals also yield meat that is higher in inflammatory omega-6 fatty acids.

You don't need to avoid meat entirely. Instead, choose organic products from animals that were raised without hormones or antibiotics, had outdoor access, and were fed a mix of grass and grain. If you don't have access to organic meat, check with your local farmer. Sometimes farms follow organic practices but cannot afford to become "certified organic" which is expensive; talk to the farmer about their practices if you don't see this label.

Sugar

There's no sugarcoating the truth: White, refined sugar is harmful to health: It spikes blood sugar, which can increase production of inflammatory cytokines (the chemical messengers involved in our immune response). Sugar produces advanced glycation end products (AGEs), substances that cause damage to cells and play a role in aging and disease. Adding to that, sugar damages teeth, robs bodies of vitamins and minerals, causes mood swings, and inhibits the immune system.

Artificial or Processed Foods

Processed foods contain many ingredients that contribute to inflammation. These include chemicals, preservatives, unhealthy fats, excess sugars, additives, artificial food dyes, refined carbohydrates, and synthetic vitamins and minerals bodies can't absorb—and more.

Eggs

According to Health Canada, eggs are a top allergen in North America and can be difficult to digest; many people are sensitive or intolerant to their protein. For people with this allergy, eggs are particularly high in inflammatory nutrients, such as omega-6 fatty acids.

Nightshade Vegetables

This family of vegetables includes tomatoes, white potatoes, eggplant, tobacco, and peppers. While many nightshades can be nutritious, they contain substances called *alkaloids*, which can cause gastrointestinal upset and aggravate inflammation in some people, particularly those who suffer from rheumatoid arthritis and osteoarthritis, headaches, lupus, kidney disease, gout, hypertension, and cancer. Nightshade foods may also leach calcium from bones and redistribute it to places where it shouldn't be, like joints, kidneys, and arteries.

FOODS THAT NOURISH AND HEAL INFLAMMATION

After learning about which foods to avoid, you might wonder what's left to eat. No worries. There is an abundance to choose from to create healthy, satisfying, and delicious meals.

As noted earlier, fruits and vegetables are anti-inflammatory all-stars. The following foods and food groups are packed with nutrients that prevent or reduce inflammation. So eat up!

Allium Vegetables

What's not to love? Onions, garlic, leeks, shallots, scallions, ramps, and chives offer a host of anti-inflammatory benefits. Onions, for example, are a rich source of the anti-inflammatory vitamin C and quercetin, which can help relieve allergy symptoms. Onions also contain *onionin A*—a molecule that targets the immune system to prevent unwanted inflammation. Garlic is no slouch either. It contains a range of sulfurous compounds that reduce inflammation throughout the body, plus it has antiviral and antibacterial properties.

Basil

Skip the aspirin. *Eugenol,* a volatile oil found in basil, inhibits the enzymes that produce inflammation, the same enzymes targeted by NSAID pain relievers.

Berries

Sweet! Blueberries, raspberries, blackberries, and strawberries are potent sources of antioxidants that combat cellular damage and inhibit the enzymes that promote inflammation.

Bone Broth

Comfort in a bowl. Bone broth (Basic Chicken Broth, page 93), prepared with organic animal bones, simmered for at least several hours, contains *glycine, proline, and arginine*—esssential amino acids. It also helps support the digestive tract by bringing digestive juices to the gut, and reduces joint pain.

Coconut Oil and Extra-Virgin Olive Oil

Remember, don't fear healthy fats. Coconut oil is a healthy, saturated fat that is especially high in lauric acid, which enriches brain function and the immune system. It's easily digested and used immediately for energy, rather than being stored as fat. Extra-virgin olive oil contains numerous polyphenols that reduce the chemical messengers and enzymes that lead to inflammation.

Cruciferous Vegetables

Lending crucial crunch, this vegetable family includes broccoli, Brussels sprouts, cabbage, cauliflower, and kale. These vegetables have special sulfur-containing phytonutrients that help the liver filter toxins and neutralize carcinogens. Studies also show that eating these veggies lowers inflammation levels in the body.

Dark Leafy Greens

Both delicious and versatile, these vegetables contain the antioxidant vitamins A, C, E, and K, which help combat cellular damage that can contribute to inflammation. They're also great sources of anti-inflammatory omega-3 fatty acids and B vitamins, which help manage stress and nourish the nervous system.

Dill

This aromatic herb helps neutralize carcinogens, and is helpful in treating digestive problems like gas, indigestion, and constipation.

Fennel

This sweet vegetable contains a number of anti-inflammatory phyto-nutrients, but is especially high in a compound called *anethole*. This phytonutrient has anti-inflammatory and anti-cancer properties, and works to shut down the signaling process that triggers inflammation. Fennel also contains antioxidants and immune-boosting nutrients.

Fish

Wild salmon, sardines, anchovies, mackerel, and halibut are wonderful sources of anti-inflammatory omega-3 fatty acids. Salmon, in particular, is high in two omega-3s called EPA and DHA, which help our bodies produce anti-inflammatory molecules. While looking out for your health with healthy food choices, remember to look out for the oceans' health, too. Choose seafood that is sustainably caught.

Ginger

Spice things up. This spicy root contains anti-inflammatory compounds called *gingerols*, which inhibit pro-inflammatory molecules. Ginger is used to treat a wide variety of conditions, including digestive issues, nausea, motion sickness, arthritis, headaches, colds, and flus.

Gluten-Free Grains

Gluten-free does not mean grain-free. Grains such as quinoa, brown rice, and millet play a unique role in an anti-inflammatory diet. Quinoa is a complete plant-based source of protein, which means it has the same amino acids found in animal products. It's also a rich source of magnesium, a relaxant mineral that reduces inflammation, and the anti-inflammatory vitamin E. Brown rice is another grain high in magnesium, along with the antioxidant selenium, which helps detoxify and protect cells from damage.

Natural Sweeteners

Go natural. While refined white sugars are inflammatory, there are a couple of natural sweeteners that can be used in an anti-inflammatory diet. Raw honey is rich in healing amino acids, digestive enzymes, and antiviral constituents. This means it helps enhance the immune system. Maple syrup is rich in antioxidants, plus it's high in zinc, another important nutrient for the immune system. Of course, the use of natural sugars is completely optional if you'd prefer to avoid sweeteners entirely.

Nuts and Seeds

Snack on. These contain a wide range of healthy fats, protein, and fiber. Walnuts, hemp, chia, and flaxseed are particularly high in omega-3 fatty acids that help combat inflammation.

Pineapple

Juicy! The core and stem of this tropical fruit contains a substance called *bromelain,* which reduces inflammation and helps us digest protein.

Root Vegetables

Earthy and satisfying, carrots, sweet potatoes, parsnips, turnips, celery root, rutabaga, and beets are all anti-inflammatory and antioxidant powerhouses. For example, both carrots and sweet potatoes are rich sources of vitamin A, which helps nourish the mucosal cells in the digestive tract, aids vision, boosts the immune system, and keeps skin healthy. Sweet potatoes contain *anthocyanin pigments* and beets are full of compounds called *betalains,* which both reduce the production of inflammatory enzymes.

Sustainable, Organic Meat

Meat is not off limits. Chicken and turkey are both high in protein, which is essential for healing and repairing inflammation. These animal products are also rich in B vitamins, particularly B_{12}, a key nutrient for the nervous system that is found rarely in plants.

Turmeric

Flavorful healing. Turmeric's anti-inflammatory power stems from its high levels of *curcumin,* which can help reduce inflammation associated with inflammatory bowel disease, arthritis, cystic fibrosis, and cancer.

Winter Squashes

Beautiful to behold, winter squashes contain high amounts of vitamins C and A, similar to root vegetables. They also contain special compounds called *cucurbitacins,* which inhibit the enzymes that lead to inflammation.

FOOD ALLERGIES, INTOLERANCES, AND SENSITIVITIES

Confused about the differences? The following should clear up any questions you have.

What Happens When . . . ?

FOOD ALLERGY: A food allergy involves an *immediate and acute immune reaction* to a food after it's eaten. Symptoms can range from a mild rash to severe anaphylaxis, where your throat swells up and you need emergency hospital treatment.

FOOD INTOLERANCE OR SENSITIVITY: This occurs when you have a reaction to certain foods, but the *immune system is not involved*. Food intolerances are often the result of flawed digestion. Our digestive tract has a special barrier that absorbs beneficial nutrients and filters out dangerous ones.

The Top Eight Allergens

1. Eggs
2. Fish
3. Milk
4. Peanuts
5. Shellfish
6. Soy
7. Tree nuts
8. Wheat

ALL RECIPES IN THIS COOKBOOK ARE DAIRY-FREE, EGG-FREE, GLUTEN-FREE, PEANUT-FREE, SHELLFISH-FREE, SOY-FREE, AND WHEAT-FREE. Some recipes contain tree nuts or fish, but you'll also find substitution tips that provide a non-allergenic alternative.

At the end of the day, we all have unique bodies and are managing different health issues. Your dietary needs will vary, depending on what you are experiencing right now. Listen to your body and modify this anti-inflammatory diet as needed. If you have a reaction every time you eat blueberries, it doesn't matter that they're on the "Enjoy" list—cross them off your list! (Though you might want to experiment with organic

FOOD LISTS
for the Anti-Inflammatory Diet

The list of foods you can enjoy on an anti-inflammatory diet is extensive, so you'll have plenty to choose from. However, foods affect each of us differently: Some may cause a reaction in certain people but not in others.

The following are controversial foods because they are linked to inflammation but also have numerous health benefits:

CITRUS. The acidity of citrus foods can aggravate inflammation in some instances but exert strong anti-inflammatory effects in others.

EGGS. If you're not allergic to eggs, then organic pastured eggs are a great source of protein, vitamin D, omega-3 fatty acids, and B vitamins—especially *choline*, which is essential to the nervous system and for producing neurotransmitters.

NIGHTSHADES. For people who are not sensitive to nightshades, this vegetable family offers numerous health benefits. For example, tomatoes contain the cancer-fighting and bone-building antioxidant *lycopene*, while eggplants are high in a special nutrient called *nasunin*, an antioxidant that fights cellular damage and boosts circulation. Peppers contain a range of antioxidants like vitamins A and C.

ENJOY

NOTE: Foods marked with an asterisk (*) are particularly powerful at fighting inflammation.

DARK LEAFY GREENS

Arugula*	Mustard greens
Collard greens*	Romaine
Kale*	Spinach*
Lettuces	Swiss chard
Mizuna	

ROOT VEGETABLES

Beets*	Rutabaga
Carrots	Sweet potatoes*
Celery root	Turnips
Kohlrabi	Yams*
Parsnips	

WINTER SQUASHES

Acorn	Kabocha
Butternut*	Pumpkin*
Delicata	Spaghetti
Hubbard	

FATS AND OILS

Avocado	Flaxseed oil*
Camelina oil	Ghee (if
Coconut oil*	tolerated)
Extra-virgin olive oil*	Hemp oil

NUTS AND SEEDS

Almonds	Hemp seeds*
Brazil nuts	Macadamia nuts
Cashews	Pumpkin seeds
Chia seeds*	Sesame seeds
Flaxseed	Walnuts*

GRAINS

Amaranth	Quinoa*
Brown rice*	Sorghum
Buckwheat*	Teff
Millet	Wild rice

BEANS AND LEGUMES

Adzuki beans	Kidney lentils
Black beans*	Lima beans
Chickpeas	Navy beans
(if tolerated)	Split peas

FRUIT

Apples	Lemon
Banana	Mango
Blackberries	Nectarines
Blueberries*	Peaches
Cherries	Pineapple
Kiwi	Strawberries

ALLIUM VEGETABLES

Chives	Scallions
Garlic*	Shallots
Onions*	

CRUCIFEROUS VEGETABLES

Broccoli*	Cauliflower*
Brussels sprouts	Kale
Cabbage*	

HERBS AND SPICES

Basil*	Ginger*
Cinnamon*	Oregano
Cloves*	Rosemary
Cumin	Sage
Dill	Turmeric*
Fennel seeds	

ANIMAL PRODUCTS

Anchovies	Mackerel
Bone broth*	Salmon*
Chicken	Sardines*
Halibut	Trout
Lamb	Turkey

SWEETENERS

Coconut sugar	Raw honey
Maple syrup	Stevia
Molasses	

AVOID

FATS AND OILS

Corn oil	Rapeseed oil
Margarine	Soybean oil
Peanut oil	Vegetable oil

NUTS AND SEEDS

Peanuts

GRAINS

Barley	Kamut
Bulgur	Semolina
Corn	Spelt
Couscous	Triticale
Farina	Wheat
Farro	

SOY BEANS

FRUIT

Citrus fruits:	Pomelo
Clementine	Satsuma
Grapefruit	Tangelo
Orange	Tangerine

NIGHTSHADE VEGETABLES

Eggplant	Tomatoes
Peppers	White potatoes
Tobacco	

ANIMAL PRODUCTS

Butter	Eggs
Cheese	Feedlot animal
Cottage	products
cheese	Ice cream
Cream cheese	Yogurt
Dairy	

SWEETENERS

Brown sugar	High-fructose
Corn syrup	corn syrup
Golden syrup	Icing sugar
	White sugar

blueberries, as the reaction could be a result of a pesticide on the fruit, rather than the fruit itself.)

It's helpful to keep a food diary while on this elimination diet—write down everything you eat, the time you consume it, and whether you notice any physical symptoms before, during, or after eating.

If you experience a reaction to food groups on the "Foods to Avoid" list (particularly the controversial foods like eggs and nightshades), then don't include them in your diet. But if you can tolerate these foods, definitely incorporate them as part of your healthful, unique diet.

SHOPPING GUIDELINES

There are a few other considerations to keep in mind when shopping and cooking on this diet:

CHOOSE ORGANIC WHEN POSSIBLE. Organic foods don't contain synthetic pesticides and toxins that threaten our health. However, organic food can be expensive. The Environmental Working Group publishes the *Shoppers Guide to Pesticides in Produce*, which contains a list of the 15 cleanest and 12 dirtiest fruits and vegetables (see Appendix B, page 189). Start by purchasing organic produce to replace those found on the "Dirty Dozen" list, while choosing conventional produce that has fewer pesticide residues.

BUY LOCAL, SEASONAL PRODUCE. The average meal travels almost 1,500 miles from farm to plate. Many people have become accustomed to eating blueberries in January and butternut squash in July, but those are not seasonal in certain climates at those times. They are fare that comes from far away and lose freshness, quality, and nutritional density. Don't forget that Mother Nature is a smart cookie—providing the precise nutrients needed to support health during each season. Plus, local and seasonal foods taste better, and are often less expensive.

STORE FOOD APPROPRIATELY. Proper food storage retains nutrients, reduces waste, and helps food last longer. This means you not only obtain the utmost benefit of a food's anti-inflammatory properties, but you'll also save some cash.

OPT FOR BPA-FREE CANNED GOODS. Tin cans full of beans or vegetables can be helpful timesavers when you need to get dinner on the table. Many canned goods are lined with bisphenol-A (BPA), a known disruptor of the endocrine system. Choose cans that have a "BPA-Free" label. Otherwise, choose frozen instead.

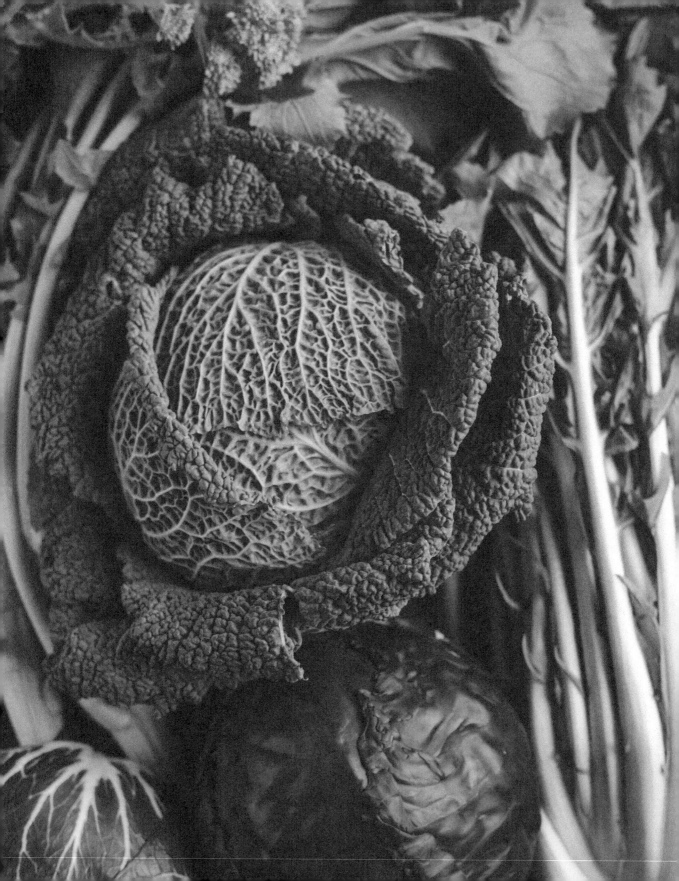

GIVING YOUR BODY A THREE-WEEK BREAK

2

It's time. If you've been dealing with aches and pains, eating poorly for whatever reason, or are simply ready for a tune-up, give your body a three-week break.

Following a temporary elimination diet removes the anti-inflammatory irritants that are damaging your health, and helps you transition to a healthier lifestyle.

This elimination diet is unique because the recipes contain only five main ingredients, which allows you to easily prepare wholesome, anti-inflammatory meals at home in a snap. Plus, simpler meals and fewer ingredients mean your pancreas won't need to produce as many enzymes to digest it all—and that lightens the load on your digestive tract and improves overall gut health.

It's important to know that the foods and recipes in this elimination plan can also be consumed long after the three weeks are over. If you're dealing with a chronic condition, or would like to prevent chronic inflammation from happening in the future, anti-inflammatory foods need to become a consistent part of your life. I aim to create recipes that are delicious and varied, as well as healthful, so you don't feel like you're missing out on anything. I won't be surprised if you'll want to keep these menu items in rotation on your table in the months to come.

SETTING YOURSELF UP FOR SUCCESS

Cooking from scratch is infinitely easier when you're organized and prepared. Here are a few of my favorite ways to transform your healthy eating intentions into concrete actions.

Tips and Tricks to Make Your Day Easier

PREPARE VEGETABLES IN ADVANCE. Chopping ingredients can be a chore. Spend a few hours each week washing, chopping, and storing all the ingredients you need for each week's recipes.

BATCH COOK ON WEEKENDS. Anti-inflammatory eating is even easier when you've got a few premade meals in the refrigerator or freezer. Make a large batch of soup, cook a large pot of grains you can pair with meals throughout the week, and throw a batch of chili in the slow cooker. If you love smoothies in the morning, prepare a week's worth of smoothie kits; simply split your greens, fruit, and nuts or seeds into individual portions, then freeze them in jars. Then, in the morning, all you'll have to do is toss your ingredients into a blender, along with the liquid, and breakfast is served.

BUY SUPERMARKET SHORTCUTS. It's not always realistic to prepare every ingredient from scratch. Buy organic, prewashed salad greens, purchase precut fresh veggies, or buy premade guacamole or hummus. The prepared options are often more expensive, but if they help you stick to your anti-inflammatory goals, then it's money well spent.

USE LEFTOVERS. There's no need to prepare a new recipe for every meal—that takes a lot of time and effort, and can lead to food waste. Consume meals repeatedly throughout the week, or double favorite recipes and freeze for another time. If you become bored, think of creative ways to repurpose food: for example, take last night's burger, crumble it up, and transform it into a taco salad for lunch.

GET THE WHOLE FAMILY INVOLVED. If you live with other people, ask them to help with preparing ingredients and cooking meals. This will speed the process and make it more enjoyable. Throw on some tunes to raise the fun factor!

The Anti-Inflammatory Pantry

A well-stocked pantry is part of organizing your kitchen and easing meal preparation. Keep the following items in stock, as you'll use them regularly in cooking the recipes in this book.

NUTS AND SEEDS

- Almonds
- Cashews
- Chia seeds
- Flaxseed
- Hemp seeds
- Pumpkin seeds
- Sunflower seeds
- Walnuts

FATS AND OILS

- Coconut oil
- Extra-virgin olive oil
- Hemp or flaxseed oil (refrigerate these)

DRIED HERBS AND SPICES

- Basil
- Cinnamon
- Coriander
- Cumin
- Dill
- Fennel
- Ginger
- Oregano
- Rosemary
- Sage
- Salt
- Thyme
- Turmeric

GRAINS AND FLOURS

- Brown rice
- Brown rice pasta
- Buckwheat
- Buckwheat noodles
- Millet
- Quinoa
- Rice noodles
- Rice paper wrappers

FROZEN FOODS

- Greens
- Mango
- Mixed berries
- Peas
- Pineapple

BEANS AND LEGUMES

- Black beans
- Chickpeas
- Kidney beans
- Lentils, brown
- Lentils, green
- Lentils, red

ANTI-INFLAMMATORY DIET
PANTRY SUBSTITUTIONS

REMOVE THIS . . .	REPLACE WITH . . .
Peanuts	Almonds, Brazil nuts, cashews, chia seeds, hemp seeds, macadamia nuts, pecans, pumpkin seeds, sesame seeds, sunflower seeds, walnuts
Barley, kamut, rye, spelt, wheat	Brown rice, buckwheat, millet, quinoa, wild rice
White or whole-wheat flour	Almond flour, arrowroot flour, brown rice flour, buckwheat flour, chickpea flour, millet flour
Soy sauce	Coconut aminos
Corn oil, peanut oil, rapeseed (canola) oil, soybean oil, vegetable oil	Coconut oil, extra-virgin olive oil
White sugar	Coconut sugar, maple syrup, raw honey
Canned tomatoes	Canned butternut squash, canned pumpkin
Iodized salt	Coarse salt, Himalayan sea salt, kosher salt
White or whole-wheat pasta	Brown rice pasta, gluten-free buckwheat noodles, rice noodles

Kitchen Equipment and Tools

So you've stocked the pantry; now it's time to take stock of your tools. Having the right equipment eases meal preparation and saves time. As the ingredients for these recipes are simple, so is the list of equipment needed. You likely already have and use most items on this list. If not, the items needed are not specialized or expensive—consider adding them to your arsenal.

- Good-quality chef's knife
- Paring knife
- Cutting board
- Measuring cups and spoons
- A few large pots and pans with lids
- Skillet or sauté pan
- Baking sheet
- Glass or ceramic ovenproof cookware
- Large stirring spoons
- Spatula
- Blender
- Food processor
- Spice grinder, or a mortar and pestle
- Mixing bowls
- Parchment paper
- Steamer basket

THE THREE-WEEK MENU PLAN

Just to review: The goal of this temporary elimination diet is to remove anti-inflammatory irritants that are damaging to your health, and help you transition to a healthier lifestyle.

There are plenty of good meals to look forward to in the next few weeks. Best of all, they're allergen-friendly and safe for even the most sensitive immune systems. *These recipes exclude almost all of the common allergens that can commonly cause a reaction*, and the few exceptions offer substitutions that are equally tasty.

We're keeping it simple. Each recipe has just five main ingredients, but in these recipes, we're not counting salt, cooking oil, or water as part of the five. Salt and oil are pantry staples, and water comes out of the tap, so using these ingredients doesn't involve any extra prep or effort. However, any other spice, herb, plant, or animal food counts.

My motto is, "Cook once; eat at least twice." To make your life easier, you'll see a number of leftovers or repeats throughout the menu plans, which will significantly cut down your prep and cooking time. You can thank me later with a batch of Strawberry Jam Thumbprint Cookies (page 166).

Over the next three weeks, remember to listen to your body. Focus on eating when you truly are hungry, and consume foods you enjoy. Switch things up in the plans as you see fit. If it's too cold on Monday morning for a smoothie, have Tuesday's oatmeal. Don't love kale? Use spinach in your stew. Just remember to swap one anti-inflammatory food for another nutritious anti-inflammatory food—not ginger root for cupcakes!

It's equally important to nourish your body in non-nutritional ways. Self-care plays a crucial role in healing, too. Take the time to rest and relax while you're following these plans, and participate in activities you enjoy. If you need help, ask for it from those you love and who love you.

WEEK ONE MENU PLAN

The hardest part of getting started is actually getting started. So put one foot in front of the other, and take it meal by meal.

If you're unfamiliar with healthy eating or anti-inflammatory foods, or are insecure about your cooking skills, the first week might be challenging. That's why this week's recipes include comfort food favorites like Tasty Fish Tacos with Pineapple Salsa (page 124), Quinoa Flatbread Pizza (page 119), and Brown Rice Pasta with Creamy Carrot "Marinara" (page 116) to help ease you into the routine. Thankfully, five-ingredient recipes make the entire cooking process easy and convenient!

For those of you who have previously experimented with clean eating, this week will probably go by without a hitch.

On your "to do" list this week:

PREP AS MUCH AS YOU CAN BEFORE THE WEEK BEGINS. If possible, ease yourself into the week by cooking the first two or three days' food on the weekend.

PAY SPECIAL ATTENTION TO HOW YOU FEEL AFTER EATING. Notice whether you experience any reactions to any foods. It helps to keep a food diary for the week, and write down your symptoms at the end of each day.

BEGIN EACH DAY WITH FIVE TO TEN DEEP BREATHS. You'll be surprised how this simple meditation can bring life-sustaining oxygen to your tissues, relax your body and mind, and reduce stress levels.

WEEK 1

WEEKLY MENU

MONDAY

Breakfast: Tropical Green Smoothie (page 55)

Lunch: Slow-Cooker Vegan Split Pea Soup (page 85)

Dinner: Brown Rice Pasta with Creamy Carrot "Marinara" (page 116)

TUESDAY

Breakfast: Avocado Toast with Greens (page 52)

Lunch: Brown Rice Pasta with Creamy Carrot "Marinara" (leftovers)

Dinner: Whitefish Chowder (page 126)

WEDNESDAY

Breakfast: "Choose Your Adventure" Chia Breakfast Pudding (page 62)

Lunch: Slow-Cooker Vegan Split Pea Soup (leftovers)

Dinner: Quinoa Flatbread Pizza (page 119)

THURSDAY

Breakfast: Strawberry Sunshine Smoothie (page 59)

Lunch: Whitefish Chowder (leftovers)

Dinner: Baby Bok Choy Stir-Fry (page 109)

FRIDAY

Breakfast: "Choose Your Adventure" Chia Breakfast Pudding (leftovers)

Lunch: Baby Bok Choy Stir-Fry (leftovers)

Dinner: Buckwheat-Vegetable Polenta (page 118)

SATURDAY

Breakfast: Blueberry-Millet Breakfast Bake (page 60)

Lunch: Buckwheat-Vegetable Polenta (leftovers)

Dinner: Tasty Fish Tacos with Pineapple Salsa (page 124)

SUNDAY

Breakfast: Blueberry-Millet Breakfast Bake (leftovers)

Lunch: Poached Chicken Wraps (page 157)

Dinner: Classic Butternut Squash Soup (page 88)

SNACKS

Pick one to two snacks per day. If you aren't hungry between meals, don't feel obligated to snack.

- Piece of fruit
- Handful of nuts or seeds
- Mug of herbal tea or bone broth (Basic Chicken Broth, page 93)
- Baked Zucchini Chips (page 71)
- No-Bake Chocolate Chip Granola Bars (page 70)
- Crudités with Roasted Fennel and Sunflower Seed Pesto* (page 179)

WEEK ONE SHOPPING LIST

CANNED AND BOTTLED ITEMS

- Applesauce, unsweetened (4 cups)
- Broth, vegetable (16 cups)
- Coconut milk, full fat (12 cups)
- Pineapple, chunks (1½ cups)

FROZEN FOODS

- Mango (1 cup)
- Pineapple (1 cup)
- Strawberries (2½ cups)

MEAT, FISH, AND POULTRY

- Chicken breasts, boneless skinless (2 [4-ounce])
- White fish, skinless and firm, such as cod or halibut (2¼ pounds)

PANTRY ITEMS

- Basil, dried
- Buckwheat (6 cups)
- Cashews (3 cups)
- Chia seeds (2 cups)
- Cinnamon, ground
- Coconut, shredded, unsweetened (⅓ cup)
- Cumin, ground
- Cranberries, dried (1 cup)
- Hemp seeds (1¼ cups)
- Honey, raw (⅓ cup)
- Millet (4 cups)
- Nuts, various, for snacking
- Olive oil, extra-virgin
- Oil, coconut
- Oregano, dried

- Pecans (1½ cups)
- Rosemary, dried
- Salt
- Sea salt
- Spaghetti, brown rice, 12-ounce package (2)
- Split peas, green or yellow (5 cups)
- Sunflower seed butter (⅓ cup)
- Sunflower seeds (¾ cup)
- Syrup, maple (1 cup)
- Thyme, dried
- Turmeric, ground
- Quinoa, dry (1½ cups)

PRODUCE

- Arugula (2 cups)
- Avocado, ripe (1)
- Basil, fresh (1 small bunch)
- Blueberries (4 cups; or frozen)
- Bok choy, baby, (24 heads)
- Butternut squash, large (2)
- Carrots, large (10)
- Carrots, medium (14)
- Celery (4 stalks)
- Crudités, various, for snacking
- Dill, fresh (1 small bunch)
- Fennel, bulbs (2)
- Fruit, various, for snacking
- Garlic, cloves (20)
- Ginger, fresh (6-inch piece)
- Kale (2 bunch)
- Lemons (4)
- Limes (2)
- Onion, red, small (1)
- Onions, yellow, large (2)
- Onions, yellow, medium (2)
- Potatoes, sweet (10)
- Romaine lettuce (2 heads)
- Spinach (21 cups)
- Zucchini, medium (6)

OTHER

- Bread, gluten-free (2 slices)
- Brown rice, cooked (6 cups)
- Chocolate chips, dairy-free (¼ cup)
- Rice paper wrappers (10)

WEEK TWO MENU PLAN

After one week, you might already feel great—with more energy and concentration, and with fewer aches and pains. That's amazing! Congratulate yourself and prepare to keep up the good work.

If you feel exactly the same as when you started, or even a little worse, don't despair. Each person will experience this plan differently, and no result, or even a negative result, doesn't mean the plan isn't working. Depending on your individual health background and needs, your journey might take a little more time.

Sometimes, when we begin to support health with nourishing, anti-inflammatory foods, our bodies begin to release the toxins they've been holding onto for so long. This can lead to some uncomfortable symptoms like digestive problems, headaches, itchiness, skin rashes, acne, joint pain, grumpiness, and more. This is real and it's called a Jarisch-Herxheimer reaction, or "die-off" reaction. It's normal and— if you continue to eat healthily—temporary.

On your "to do" list this week:

CONTINUE WITH YOUR DAILY FOOD DIARY. Track symptoms, prep food, and take cleansing breaths.

ADD DAILY EXERCISE ACTIVITY. Choose something you already know and love, or try something new! I recommend gentle exercise at this point, like walking, hatha yoga, swimming, or an easy bike ride.

FOCUS ON THE POSITIVE. Make a list of the good things that have happened to you since beginning your anti-inflammatory diet, or write down all the things you are grateful for (family, a warm bed, food in the refrigerator, etc.).

WEEKLY MENU

MONDAY

Breakfast: Tropical Green Smoothie (page 55)

Lunch: Classic Butternut Squash Soup (leftover from Week One)

Dinner: Coconut Chicken Curry (page 161)

TUESDAY

Breakfast: Maple-Tahini Oatmeal (page 53)

Lunch: Coconut Chicken Curry (leftovers)

Dinner: Home-Style Red Lentil Stew (page 114)

WEDNESDAY

Breakfast: "Quick Greens and Cauliflower Bowl (page 64)

Lunch: Gluten-Free Ramen "To Go" (page 84)

Dinner: Sesame-Tuna with Asparagus (page 131)

THURSDAY

Breakfast: Butternut Squash Smoothie (page 54)

Lunch: Home-Style Red Lentil Stew (leftovers)

Dinner: Slow-Cooker Chicken Alfredo (page 153)

FRIDAY

Breakfast: Tropical Green Smoothie (page 55)

Lunch: Slow-Cooker Chicken Alfredo (leftovers)

Dinner: Homemade Avocado Sushi (page 113)

SATURDAY

Breakfast: Maple-Cinnamon Granola (page 65)

Lunch: Cream of Broccoli Soup (page 87)

Dinner: Root Vegetable Loaf (page 102) with Cumin-Roasted Cauliflower (page 79)

SUNDAY

Breakfast: Maple-Cinnamon Granola (leftovers)

Lunch: Cream of Broccoli Soup (leftovers)

Dinner: Vegetable Spring Roll Wraps (page 107)

SNACKS

Pick one to two snacks per day. If you aren't hungry between meals, don't feel obligated to snack.

- Crispy Roasted Chickpeas* (page 77)
- Carrot and Raisin Salad* (page 95)
- Half an avocado (sprinkled with sea salt)
- 1 or 2 Medjool dates, sliced open and spread with nut or seed butter
- Apple topped with nut or seed butter
- Crudités with Creamy Lentil Dip* (page 184), or purchased hummus or guacamole

WEEK TWO SHOPPING LIST

CANNED AND BOTTLED ITEMS

- Butternut squash purée (3 cups)
- Coconut milk (7 cups)
- Tahini (1 cup)

FROZEN FOODS

- Mango (2 cups)
- Pineapple (2 cups)

MEAT, FISH, AND POULTRY

- Chicken thighs, bone-in skinless (12 [2–3-ounce])
- Chicken thighs, boneless skinless (4 pounds)
- Tuna steaks (4 [4-ounce])

PANTRY ITEMS

- Cashews (4 cups)
- Chickpeas, dried (1 cup)
- Cinnamon, ground
- Coriander, ground
- Cumin, ground
- Curry powder
- Dates, Medjool, for snacking
- Garlic powder
- Hemp seeds (½ cup)
- Lentils, green or brown (1 cup)
- Lentils, red (6 cups)
- Oats, rolled, gluten-free (11 cups)
- Olive oil, extra-virgin

- Oil, coconut (1½ cups)
- Onion powder
- Oregano, dried
- Raisins (1 cup)
- Salt
- Sea salt
- Sesame oil, toasted (3 tablespoons)
- Sesame seeds (2 tablespoons)
- Sunflower seeds (4 cups)
- Syrup, maple (2 cups)
- Quinoa, dry (2 cups)

PRODUCE

- Apples, for snacking
- Asparagus (2 bunches)
- Avocados (6)
- Broccoli, whole (8 bunches)
- Carrots, medium (24)
- Cauliflower, florets (1½ cups)
- Cauliflower, large (2 heads)
- Cauliflower, medium (2 heads)
- Celery (8 stalks)
- Crudités, various, for snacking
- Cucumbers, small (2)
- Garlic, cloves (9)
- Ginger, fresh (2-inch piece)
- Kale, leaves (5)
- Lemons (4)
- Onions (7)
- Potatoes, sweet, large (3)
- Spinach (13 cups)
- Spinach, baby (2 cups)
- Swiss chard (6 bunches)
- Zucchini (4)

OTHER

- Coconut aminos
- Nori sheets (6)
- Rice paper wrappers (10)
- Soba noodles, cooked (½ cup)
- Vegetable broth powder (1 teaspoon)

WEEK THREE MENU PLAN

You should be feeling the difference by now and, hopefully, you're in the groove of prepping ingredients, grocery shopping, cooking, and eating. Everything should be feeling much easier than in Week One.

Keep in mind that it's impossible to completely transform your life in a few short weeks. You've made some incredible, health-affirming changes in the last 14 days and you should celebrate that. Don't be discouraged if it still feels hard; lasting change takes time. It took me years to stay on a steady anti-inflammatory path. I occasionally relapsed and indulged in inflammatory foods before getting back on track permanently—and now the junky foods I used to eat all the time don't tempt me in the least.

Feel the Craving?

As it's still early on your journey, you might be experiencing some cravings for sugar, dairy, gluten, or any other food you miss right now. Here are some tips to help deal with this:

- Make yourself a cup of tea and sit down at the table to enjoy it.
- Post notes to your cupboard or refrigerator that remind you of your uncomfortable or painful inflammatory symptoms.
- Replace your eating ritual with another activity. For example, if you're tempted to snack in front of the television each night, take a walk, read a book, or call a friend instead.
- Consume healthy, anti-inflammatory snacks such as a cup of warm almond milk sweetened with raw honey, a rice cake with hummus or guacamole, or a square of dark chocolate (85 percent cacao or higher).

On your "to do" list this week:

Take this last week to celebrate what you've achieved, and to cement healthy anti-inflammatory habits that will take you into the future.

WEEK 3

WEEKLY MENU

MONDAY

Breakfast: Strawberry Sunshine Smoothie (page 59)

Lunch: Herbed Tuna Cakes (page 138)

Dinner: Quinoa-Lentil Salad (page 97)

TUESDAY

Breakfast: Quick Greens and Cauliflower Bowl (page 64)

Lunch: Brown Rice Congee (page 142)

Dinner: Almond-Crusted Honey-Dijon Salmon with Greens (page 137)

WEDNESDAY

Breakfast: "Choose Your Adventure" Chia Breakfast Pudding (page 62)

Lunch: Brown Rice Congee (leftovers)

Dinner: Carrot-Ginger Soup (page 86)

THURSDAY

Breakfast: "Choose Your Adventure" Chia Breakfast Pudding (leftovers)

Lunch: Quinoa-Lentil Salad (leftovers)

Dinner: Yam-Bean Burgers (page 104)

FRIDAY

Breakfast: Avocado Toast with Greens (page 52)

Lunch: Carrot-Ginger Soup (leftovers)

Dinner: Sardine Donburi (page 123)

SATURDAY

Breakfast: Gluten-Free Toast with Toasted Coconut Sunbutter (page 181)

Lunch: Glorious Creamed Greens Soup (page 92)

Dinner: Yam-Bean Burgers (leftovers)

SUNDAY

Breakfast: Tropical Green Smoothie (page 55)

Lunch: Glorious Creamed Greens Soup (leftovers)

Dinner: Apple-Turkey Burgers (page 147) with Garlicky Sautéed Greens (page 99)

SNACKS

Pick one to two snacks per day. If you aren't hungry between meals, don't feel obligated to snack.

- 1 cup of any soup leftovers
- 1 or 2 pieces of Quinoa Flatbread (page 76) spread with nut butter, or purchased hummus or guacamole
- Half a steamed sweet potato mashed with coconut oil, hemp seeds, and sea salt
- Crudités with Veggie Pâté* (page 182)
- Chocolate-Avocado Pudding* (page 165)

WEEK THREE SHOPPING LIST

CANNED AND BOTTLED ITEMS

- Coconut milk (15 cups)
- Mustard, Dijon (⅓ cup)
- Sardines, canned (3 [4-ounce]) cans
- Tuna, wild, canned (2 [6-ounce]) cans

FROZEN FOODS

- Mango (1 cup)
- Pineapple (1 cup)
- Strawberries (2½ cups)

MEAT, FISH, AND POULTRY

- Bones, chicken (4 pounds)
- Turkey, ground (1 pound)

PANTRY ITEMS

- Almonds, whole (¾ cup)
- Brown rice (7 cups)
- Chia seeds (1½ cups)
- Cinnamon, ground
- Coconut, unsweetened, large-flake (1½ cups)
- Cranberries, dried (1 cup)
- Dates, Medjool (12)
- Flaxseed, ground (2 tablespoons)
- Flour, almond (¼ cup)
- Flour, chickpea (¼ cup)
- Hemp seeds (1¼ cups)
- Honey, raw (3 tablespoons)
- Lentils, green, brown, or French (2 cups)

- Oats, rolled, gluten-free (2 cups)
- Olive oil, extra-virgin
- Oil, coconut (3 tablespoons)
- Quinoa, dry (3½ cups)
- Salt
- Sea salt
- Sesame oil, toasted (½ cup)
- Sunflower seed butter (1 cup)
- Sunflower seeds (1½ cups)
- Syrup, maple (½ cup)
- Turmeric, ground

PRODUCE

- Apple (1)
- Avocados (4)
- Broccoli (2 heads)
- Carrots, medium (24)
- Cauliflower, florets (1½ cups)
- Collard greens, tightly packed (8 cups)
- Crudités, various, for snacking
- Fennel, fresh (2 bunches)
- Garlic, cloves (10)
- Ginger, fresh (10-inch piece)
- Kale, leaves (4)
- Kale, tightly packed (11 cups)
- Lemons (3)
- Onions, large (2)
- Onion, medium (1)
- Onion, red (1)
- Onions, small (2)
- Parsley, fresh (5 bunches)
- Potatoes, sweet, large (2)
- Scallions (3)
- Spinach (22 cups)
- Swiss chard (3 bunches)
- Swiss chard, tightly packed (3 cups)
- Yams, large (4)
- Zucchini (1)

OTHER

- Basic Chicken Broth (16 cups; ingredients included in shopping list)
- Bread, gluten-free (4 slices)
- Cacao powder (½ cup)
- Carrot purée (4 cups)
- Hummus, purchased, for snacking
- Navy beans, cooked (6 cups)
- Parsnips, cooked, mashed (2 cups)

A LIFESTYLE FREE OF INFLAMMATION

After following this plan for three weeks, you should feel better and be prepped to stay on the anti-inflammatory plan for continued good health. Following are some helpful, practical ways to stay on track as you continue to move forward:

1. **EAT VEGGIES WHENEVER YOU CAN.** Don't misunderstand; fruits are good for you, but it's easy to eat a crisp apple, sweet cherries, or a juicy ripe peach. Focus on eating a wide variety of nutrient-rich vegetables, particularly dark leafy greens. Toss a few handfuls into your smoothies, or cook them in soups, stews, casseroles, pasta dishes, and sauces.

2. **CONSUME MORE PLANT-BASED PROTEIN THAN ANIMAL PROTEIN.** Certain animal foods, such as bone broth and fish, are anti-inflammatory. Overall, though, excess animal foods can cause inflammation. So, focus on bulking up your diet with easily digestible plant-based pro-teins. Aim to eat no more than one meal per day with animal products.

3. **DRINK WATER AND HERBAL TEAS.** Ditch the coffee, soda, alcohol, and sugar-laden juices for at least eight cups of water per day. Water is an essential beverage that sweeps toxins away, lubricates the digestive tract, reduces pain, and minimizes allergy and asthma symptoms. If plain water sounds boring, spruce it up with slices of cucumber or lemon, berries, or herbs like mint or lavender.

4. **SCHEDULE STRESS-REDUCTION ACTIVITIES IN YOUR CALENDAR.** Anti-inflammatory nutrition will be less effective if you are tense, worried, or angry. Our emotions and thoughts play a huge role in our health and stress can impact our ability to regulate our immune system. Of course, not stressing out is easier said than done. It helps immensely if you book stress relief into your calendar as an appointment *and keep it*, much like you would an appointment with the doctor or dentist. I like to set aside 30 minutes per day. Make yours of the length and at the time of day that will keep you committed.

5. **EXERCISE REGULARLY, BUT GENTLY.** Consistent physical activity helps reduce inflammation, but you don't need to run a triathlon to reap the benefits. If you're dealing with chronic pain or fatigue, it can be especially challenging to tackle an exercise routine. So keep it simple, easy, and gentle. Take a daily walk, go for a bike ride, attend a yoga class, or follow a fitness class on YouTube.

6. **MAKE SMART CHOICES WHEN EATING OUT.** Anti-inflammatory eating doesn't mean being chained to the stove. When eating out, choose a restaurant that uses fresh, whole ingredients. It will be easier to find a meal, or make a special request for one, that will accommodate your diet. Call the restaurant in advance and explain any dietary restrictions so they can prepare in advance; many restaurants today are eager to accommodate you, even if they don't already have appropriate choices on the menu, as many chefs already prepare for many types of food allergies and train servers in the menu's ingredients.

   Choose menu items packed with vegetables, plant-based proteins, or lean meat or fish, and skip the pasta, white rice, and bread. Also, don't be afraid to ask your server about ingredients, especially sauces or marinades which can be loaded with inflammatory ingredients such as gluten, dairy, or soy. A healthy meal of fish and vegetables can go from great to inflammatory if it's doused in cream sauce—but it's easy to request a drizzle of olive oil and lemon instead.

7. **DECREASE CHEMICAL EXPOSURE IN THE HOME.** Food isn't the only part of the inflammatory picture. Chemicals found in household cleaning products, cosmetics, personal care products, and sunscreens can all contribute to inflammation. Reduce your overall toxic load by replacing these products with less harmful, eco-friendly alternatives, or consider making your own. A little water, lemon, and baking soda can be amazingly effective at cleaning your home!

8. **CELEBRATE HOLIDAYS WITH A FEW SIMPLE TWEAKS.** Similar to when you eat out, holidays don't need to be a culinary nightmare. If you're up to it, offer to host family events so you can create healthy, yet familiar, anti-inflammatory fare. You don't need to make drastic changes—a simple roasted chicken served with sautéed vegetables, herb-stuffed rice, and homemade gluten-free flatbread, can be deliciously anti-inflammatory.

However, if you're attending a celebration at someone else's home, explain that you are working on your health and offer to bring an anti-inflammatory dish to share with everyone. Also, it's important to remember that the holidays are about spending time with family, not food. Suggest fun seasonal activities, like going to the beach or ice skating, that you can participate in without the need for food.

9. **SLEEP FOR SEVEN TO EIGHT HOURS PER NIGHT.** Lack of sleep is associated with higher levels of inflammation. Quality shut-eye is important because it allows us to ingrain what we've learned throughout the day, as well as repair, recharge, and regenerate body tissues. Try to go to bed at the same time every evening, so your body can regulate its sleep cycle. It also helps to slumber in a dark, cool room, and to shut off all electronic devices at least an hour before bedtime.

10. **TALK TO YOUR DOCTOR FOR TARGETED ADVICE.** Your health status is unique, and your health care team can help you devise a plan that will specifically address your individual concerns and needs. Talk to your doctor for additional information, advice, and tips about reducing or managing inflammation.

Incorporating anti-inflammatory nutrition and lifestyle changes takes practice, but like any skill, it becomes easier with time. Before you know it, you won't remember how you lived before. And, since you'll feel much better, you'll be motivated to continue on the path you created to vibrant health.

Now the fun part—let's cook!

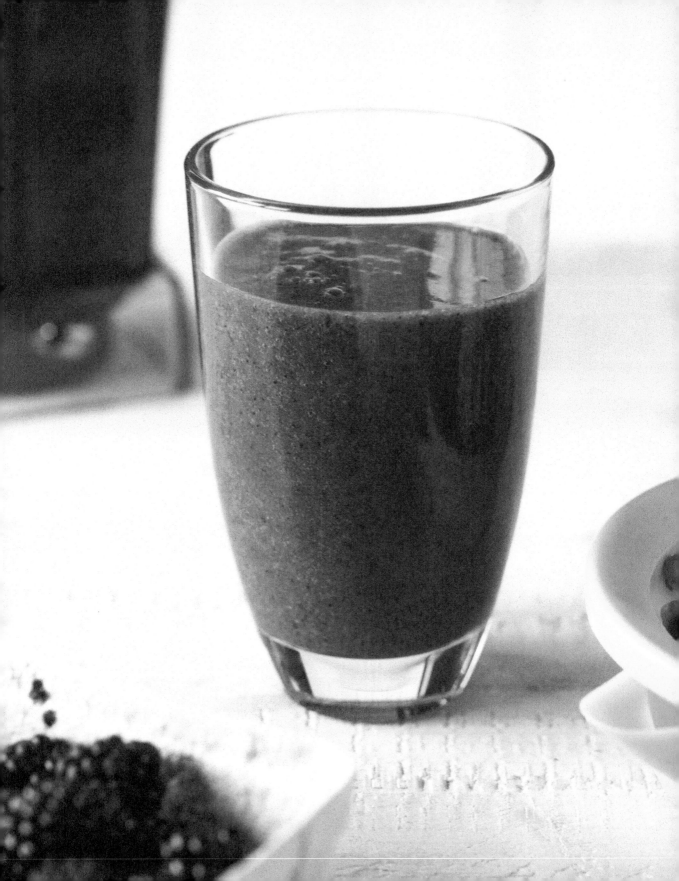

SMOOTHIES and BREAKFASTS

3

AVOCADO TOAST with GREENS

SERVES 1 · PREP TIME: 5 MINUTES · COOK TIME: 4 MINUTES

CORN FREE
DAIRY FREE
EGG FREE
GLUTEN FREE
NIGHTSHADE FREE
NUT FREE
SOY FREE
VEGAN

There are myriad ingredients you can use to top your avocado toast—sliced radishes, cucumber wedges, salsa, pesto, smoked salmon, tahini, and more—but I like to keep it lean and green with the addition of spinach. As a bonus, the healthy fats found in avocado help you better absorb the nutrients in the greens!

2 slices gluten-free bread

1 ripe avocado, halved and pitted

1½ tablespoons freshly squeezed lemon juice, plus additional as needed

⅛ teaspoon salt, plus additional as needed

2 cups lightly packed spinach leaves

1   Toast the bread.

2   Fill a medium pot with 2 inches of water and insert a steamer basket. Bring the water to a boil over high heat.

3   Into a small bowl, scoop the avocado flesh from the peel with a spoon.

4   Add the lemon juice and salt. Mash together with a fork. Taste, and adjust the seasoning with more lemon juice or salt, if necessary.

5   When the water boils, add the spinach to the steamer basket. Cover and steam for 3 to 4 minutes, or until wilted.

6   Divide the avocado mixture between the two pieces of toast. Top each with half of the wilted greens.

INGREDIENT TIP: *How can you tell if an avocado is ripe? Gently press the tip of your nose with your finger. The gentle yield of your nose to your finger is what you should feel when assessing an avocado.*

PER SERVING Calories: 589; Total Fat: 44g; Total Carbohydrates: 46g; Sugar: 18g; Fiber: 2g; Protein: 6g; Sodium: 219mg

MAPLE-TAHINI OATMEAL

SERVES 2   PREP TIME: 5 MINUTES   COOK TIME: 15 MINUTES

CORN FREE
DAIRY FREE
EGG FREE
GLUTEN FREE
NIGHTSHADE FREE
NUT FREE
SOY FREE
VEGAN

If you're not eating dairy, where do you get calcium? One answer that might not come to mind immediately: sesame seeds! These seeds are tiny but mighty, and one of the best sources of plant-based, bioavailable bone-building calcium. They are also rich in many other nutrients such as iron, zinc, magnesium, and selenium.

2 cups water

1 cup gluten-free rolled oats

⅛ teaspoon salt

⅓ cup tahini

2 tablespoons maple syrup, divided

1   In a medium pot set over medium-high heat, stir together the water, oats, and salt. Bring to a boil. Reduce the heat to low and cover. Simmer for about 10 minutes, stirring occasionally, and checking for tenderness.

2   Stir in the tahini, letting it melt into the oatmeal. Cook for 3 to 4 minutes more, or until the oatmeal is cooked through.

3   Divide the oatmeal between two bowls. Drizzle each with 1 table-spoon of maple syrup.

INGREDIENT TIP: *You can buy tahini at the grocery store, but it's also easy (and less expensive) to make your own. Roast 3 cups of sesame seeds in a 350°F oven for 8 minutes. Process the toasted seeds in a food processor until smooth and creamy. Refrigerate.*

PER SERVING Calories: 500; Total Fat: 28g; Total Carbohydrates: 55g; Sugar: 9g; Fiber: 12g; Protein: 15g; Sodium: 131mg

BUTTERNUT SQUASH SMOOTHIE

SERVES 2   PREP TIME: 5 MINUTES   COOK TIME: 0 MINUTES

CORN FREE
DAIRY FREE
EGG FREE
GLUTEN FREE
NIGHTSHADE FREE
NUT FREE
SOY FREE
VEGAN

It might seem odd to use squash as the base for a smoothie, but—trust me—this is delicious! It's smooth, creamy, and satisfying, like having a milk shake for breakfast!

2 cups butternut squash purée, frozen in ice cube trays (see Ingredient Tip)

1 cup coconut milk, plus additional as needed

¼ cup tahini

¼ cup maple syrup

1 teaspoon cinnamon

1   Release the butternut squash cubes from the ice cube trays and put them in a blender.

2   Add the coconut milk, tahini, maple syrup, and cinnamon.

3   Blend until smooth. If the consistency is too thick, thin with water or more coconut milk to achieve the desired consistency.

4   Pour into two glasses and serve.

SUBSTITUTION TIP: *Not a fan of tahini? If nut allergies aren't an issue, substitute almond butter, cashew butter, or pecan butter.*

INGREDIENT TIP: *Butternut squash purée is easy to make! Steam butternut squash cubes until tender (about 7 minutes) and purée in a food processor or blender. Store the cooked purée in jars in the freezer, or freeze in ice cube trays. If you are unable to make the purée yourself, purchase it canned (in a BPA-free can, preferably).*

PER SERVING Calories: 660; Total Fat: 48g; Total Carbohydrates: 59g; Sugar: 28g; Fiber: 11g; Protein: 10g; Sodium: 260mg

TROPICAL GREEN SMOOTHIE

SERVES 2   PREP TIME: 5 MINUTES   COOK TIME: 0 MINUTES

CORN FREE
DAIRY FREE
EGG FREE
GLUTEN FREE
NIGHTSHADE FREE
NUT FREE
SOY FREE
VEGAN

If you've never tried a green smoothie, start with this one. The mango and pineapple bring sweetness and tang, and the spinach is so mild you won't even taste it. If you like stronger greens, add kale or arugula instead. And, if you've got some protein powder in the cupboard, toss some in, too.

2½ cups spinach

1½ cups water

1 cup frozen pineapple

1 cup frozen mango

¼ cup hemp seeds

1 teaspoon grated fresh ginger

1   In a blender, combine the spinach, water, pineapple, mango, hemp seeds, and ginger. Blend until smooth.

2   Pour into two glasses and enjoy.

STORAGE TIP: *Can't finish your green smoothie? Freeze the leftovers in an ice cube tray and add the cubes to another smoothie later.*

PER SERVING Calories: 196; Total Fat: 7g; Total Carbohydrates: 29g; Sugar: 24g; Fiber: 5g; Protein: 7g; Sodium: 30mg

EAT YOUR GREENS SMOOTHIE

SERVES 1   PREP TIME: 5 MINUTES   COOK TIME: 0 MINUTES

CORN FREE
DAIRY FREE
EGG FREE
GLUTEN FREE
NIGHTSHADE FREE
NUT FREE
SOY FREE
PALEO
VEGAN

This refreshing, fiber-rich smoothie is like drinking a salad! If you want to up your greens intake, this smoothie makes it easy to do just that. The avocado and pear add sweetness; if it's not enough, toss in some honey or a Medjool date.

¾ to 1 cup water

1 cup lightly packed spinach leaves

2 kale leaves, thoroughly washed

2 romaine lettuce leaves

½ avocado

1 pear, stemmed, cored, and chopped

1   In a blender, combine the water, spinach, kale, romaine lettuce, avocado, and pear.

2   Blend until smooth and serve.

INGREDIENT TIP: *Add extra "oomph" to this smoothie with the juice and zest of one lime, along with some grated fresh ginger.*

PER SERVING Calories: 180; Total Fat: 10g; Total Carbohydrates: 23g; Sugar: 7g; Fiber: 7g; Protein: 4g; Sodium: 45mg

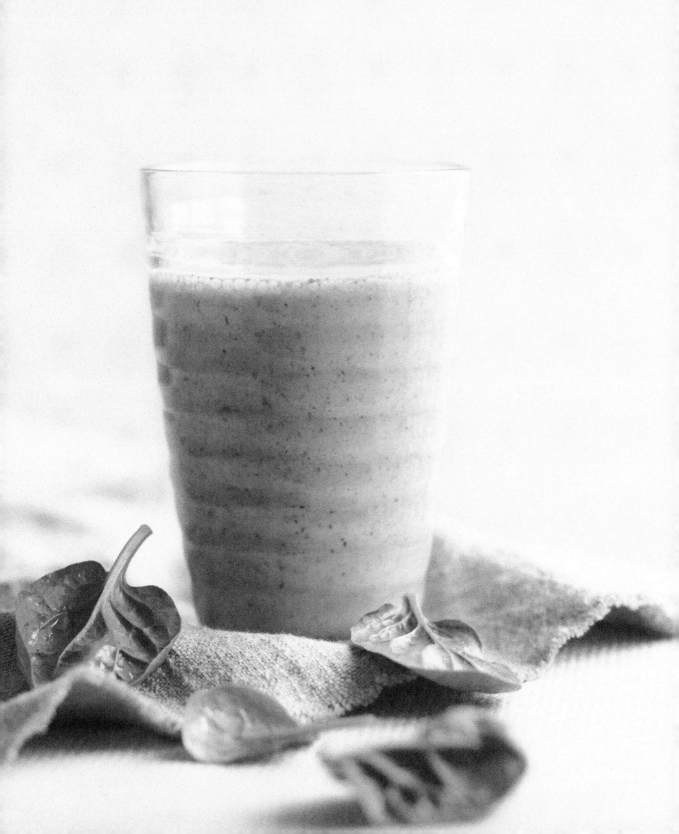

VERY BERRY SMOOTHIE

SERVES 1   PREP TIME: 5 MINUTES   COOK TIME: 0 MINUTES

CORN FREE
DAIRY FREE
EGG FREE
GLUTEN FREE
NIGHTSHADE FREE
NUT FREE
SOY FREE
VEGAN

Berries are a deliciously rich source of antioxidants, fiber, and anti-inflammatory nutrients—and a great way to start the day. I love raspberries, strawberries, and blackberries in this recipe, but you can use any berry you love. Conventional berries are sprayed with high amounts of pesticides, so choose organic whenever you can.

¾ to 1 cup water

½ cup frozen raspberries

½ cup frozen strawberries

¼ cup frozen blackberries

2 tablespoons nut butter or seed butter, such as almond butter, sunflower seed butter, tahini, etc.

1   In a blender, combine the water, raspberries, strawberries, blackberries, and nut butter.

2   Blend until smooth and serve.

INGREDIENT TIP: *Berries are at their peak during summertime. Buy extra berries from your local farmer and freeze them. You'll enjoy them all winter long (and save some cash, too!).*

PER SERVING Calories: 186; Total Fat: 9g; Total Carbohydrates: 24g; Sugar: 17g; Fiber: 5g; Protein: 4g; Sodium: 1mg

STRAWBERRY SUNSHINE SMOOTHIE

SERVES 2   PREP TIME: 5 MINUTES   COOK TIME: 0 MINUTES

CORN FREE
DAIRY FREE
EGG FREE
GLUTEN FREE
NIGHTSHADE FREE
NUT FREE
SOY FREE
VEGAN

Ground turmeric is a highly anti-inflammatory spice, but it has a strong taste. Start with just ⅛ teaspoon, and work your way up from there. Eventually, you may get to the point where you can add an entire teaspoon—and amp up the anti-inflammatory benefits!

2½ cups frozen strawberries

2 cups spinach

1¼ cups coconut milk

½ teaspoon ground cinnamon

⅛ to ¼ teaspoon
ground turmeric

1   In a blender, combine the strawberries, spinach, coconut milk, cinnamon, and turmeric. Blend until smooth.

2   Pour into two glasses and enjoy.

SUBSTITUTION TIP: *Substitute any frozen fruit or berry in this recipe—blueberries, blackberries, raspberries, cherries, apricots, or anything you prefer.*

PER SERVING Calories: 417; Total Fat: 36g; Total Carbohydrates: 26g; Sugar: 16g; Fiber: 8g; Protein: 4g; Sodium: 46mg

BLUEBERRY-MILLET BREAKFAST BAKE

SERVES 8   PREP TIME: 10 MINUTES   COOK TIME: 55 MINUTES

Millet isn't just for the birds. This mild, nutty grain is full of antioxidants and high in magnesium, a mineral that helps relax muscles. Soaking millet overnight helps it cook quickly and releases the antinutrients and enzyme inhibitors that interfere with digestion. This recipe is a crowd-pleaser for breakfast or brunch.

2 cups millet, soaked in water overnight

2 cups fresh, or frozen, blueberries

1¾ cups unsweetened applesauce

⅓ cup coconut oil, melted

2 teaspoons grated fresh ginger

1½ teaspoons ground cinnamon

1   Preheat the oven to 350°F.

2   In a fine-mesh sieve, drain and rinse the millet for 1 to 2 minutes. Transfer to a large bowl.

3   Gently fold in the blueberries, applesauce, coconut oil, ginger, and cinnamon.

4   Pour the mixture into a 9-by-9-inch casserole dish. Cover with aluminum foil.

5   Place the dish in the preheated oven and bake for 40 minutes. Remove the foil and bake for 10 to 15 minutes more, or until lightly crisp on top.

INGREDIENT TIP: *The applesauce and fruit lend a natural sweetness but if this dish isn't sweet enough, drizzle some maple syrup or raw honey on top. It's also delicious served with coconut yogurt!*

NOTE *that the Week One Plan calls for leftovers; double the quantities so you have enough for later in the week.*

PER SERVING Calories: 323; Total Fat: 13g; Total Carbohydrates: 48g; Sugar: 9g; Fiber: 6g; Protein: 6g; Sodium: 4mg

SAVORY QUINOA BREAKFAST STEW

SERVES 1   PREP TIME: 5 MINUTES   COOK TIME: 17 MINUTES

CORN FREE
DAIRY FREE
EGG FREE
GLUTEN FREE
NIGHTSHADE FREE
NUT FREE
SOY FREE
VEGAN

You're probably used to eating breakfast porridges filled with maple syrup, cinnamon, dried fruits, and nuts. While there's nothing wrong with that, a savory breakfast offers the opportunity to incorporate more vegetables into your diet. This recipe is rich in protein and fiber, which will keep you feeling full all morning long—and it's incredibly versatile. Switch up the vegetables or herbs to suit your tastes, and double and triple the quantities for a crowd (or for leftovers to eat throughout the week).

¼ cup quinoa

¾ cup water, plus additional as needed

½ small broccoli head, finely chopped

1 carrot, grated

¼ teaspoon salt

1 tablespoon chopped fresh dill

1   In a fine-mesh strainer, rinse the quinoa well.

2   In a small pot set over high heat, stir together the quinoa and water. Bring to a boil. Reduce the heat to low. Cover and cook for 5 minutes.

3   Add the broccoli, carrot, and salt. Cook for 10 to 12 minutes more, or until the quinoa is fully cooked and tender. If the stew gets too dry, add more water. This should be on the liquid side as opposed to the drier consistency of a pilaf.

4   Fold in the dill and serve.

SUBSTITUTION TIP: *Play around with different gluten-free grains. Gluten-free rolled oats, millet, buckwheat, sorghum, teff, and amaranth are all good options. You can also experiment with either keeping the grains whole or grinding them in a food processor for a thick, farina-like texture.*

PER SERVING Calories: 220; Total Fat: 3g; Total Carbohydrates: 41g; Sugar: 5g; Fiber: 7g; Protein: 10g; Sodium: 667mg

"CHOOSE YOUR ADVENTURE" CHIA BREAKFAST PUDDING

SERVES 4   PREP TIME: 5 MINUTES   COOK TIME: 0 MINUTES

CORN FREE
DAIRY FREE
EGG FREE
GLUTEN FREE
NIGHTSHADE FREE
NUT FREE
SOY FREE
VEGAN

I love this chia pudding because it's rich in calcium, protein, and anti-inflammatory omega-3 fats, and also because you can create endless variations. Start with the basic recipe and play around with the liquid, sweeteners, and other add-ins. You can even create a topping "buffet" so everyone can customize their own bowl.

¾ cup chia seeds

½ cup hemp seeds

2¼ cups coconut milk

½ cup dried cranberries

¼ cup maple syrup

1   In a medium bowl, stir together the chia seeds, hemp seeds, coconut milk, cranberries, and maple syrup, ensuring that the chia is completely mixed with the milk.

2   Cover the bowl and refrigerate overnight.

3   In the morning, stir and serve.

INGREDIENT TIP: *If you don't like the consistency of whole chia seeds, blend them with the coconut milk before adding the remaining ingredients. This will produce a smoother pudding.*

NOTE *that the Week One and Week Three Plans call for leftovers; double the quantities so you have enough for later in those weeks.*

ADDITIONAL INGREDIENT OPTIONS:

Nondairy milk: almond milk, cashew milk, rice milk, sesame milk, hemp milk, oat milk

Dried fruit: raisins, blueberries, apricots, dates, goji berries, apples

Grains: swap ¼ cup of buckwheat groats for the chia seeds

Sweeteners: raw honey, stevia, or coconut sugar

Make it fancy: vanilla, cinnamon, dairy-free chocolate chips or cacao nibs, walnuts, pumpkin seeds, ground ginger

Get fresh: fresh fruit

PER SERVING Calories: 483; Total Fat: 41g; Total Carbohydrates: 25g; Sugar: 17g; Fiber: 6g; Protein: 9g; Sodium: 22mg

QUICK GREENS and CAULIFLOWER BOWL

SERVES 1   PREP TIME: 5 MINUTES   COOK TIME: 5 MINUTES

CORN FREE
DAIRY FREE
EGG FREE
GLUTEN FREE
NIGHTSHADE FREE
NUT FREE
SOY FREE
VEGAN

Cruciferous vegetables in the morning? Well, why not? These hot, tender-crisp vegetables make for a light, nourishing breakfast that is ready in minutes. If you'd like to add extra protein, toss in a handful of beans, or flake in a few chunks of leftover salmon.

4 kale leaves, thoroughly washed and chopped

1½ cups cauliflower florets

½ avocado, chopped

1 teaspoon freshly squeezed lemon juice

1 teaspoon extra-virgin olive oil

Pinch salt

1   Fill a medium pot with 2 inches of water and insert a steamer basket. Bring to a boil over high heat.

2   Add the kale and cauliflower to the basket. Cover and steam for 5 minutes.

3   Transfer the vegetables to a medium bowl. Toss with the avocado, lemon juice, olive oil, and salt.

MAKE AHEAD TIP: *Chop the cauliflower and kale the night before, place them in the steamer basket, and refrigerate overnight. In the morning, they'll be ready to cook when you are.*

PER SERVING Calories: 317; Total Fat: 25g; Total Carbohydrates: 24g; Sugar: 4g; Fiber: 12g; Protein: 7g; Sodium: 236mg

MAPLE-CINNAMON GRANOLA

SERVES 8 TO 10   PREP TIME: 15 MINUTES   COOK TIME: 35 TO 40 MINUTES

CORN FREE
DAIRY FREE
EGG FREE
GLUTEN FREE
NIGHTSHADE FREE
NUT FREE
SOY FREE
VEGAN

Skip the expensive, store-bought granolas and make this one at home instead. Once you have this simple recipe down, it can be embellished with additional fruits like dried apple or cranberry; more spices such as ground ginger, cardamom, or cloves; dried coconut; or nuts (pecans are especially good).

4 cups gluten-free rolled oats

1½ cups sunflower seeds

½ cup maple syrup

½ cup coconut oil

1½ teaspoons ground cinnamon

1   Preheat the oven to 325°F.

2   Line two baking sheets with parchment paper.

3   In a large bowl, stir together the oats, sunflower seeds, maple syrup, coconut oil, and cinnamon. Stir well so the oats and seeds are evenly coated with the syrup, oil, and cinnamon.

4   Divide the granola mixture evenly between the two sheets.

5   Place the sheets in the preheated oven and bake for 35 to 40 minutes, stirring every 10 minutes so everything browns evenly.

6   Cool completely, then store in large glass jars with tight-fitting lids.

SUBSTITUTION TIP: *If you like your granola chunkier and clumpy, use melted honey instead of maple syrup.*

NOTE *that the Week Two Plan calls for leftovers; double the quantities so you have enough for later in the week.*

PER SERVING Calories: 400; Total Fat: 22g; Total Carbohydrates: 47g; Sugar: 12g; Fiber: 6g; Protein: 9g; Sodium: 3mg

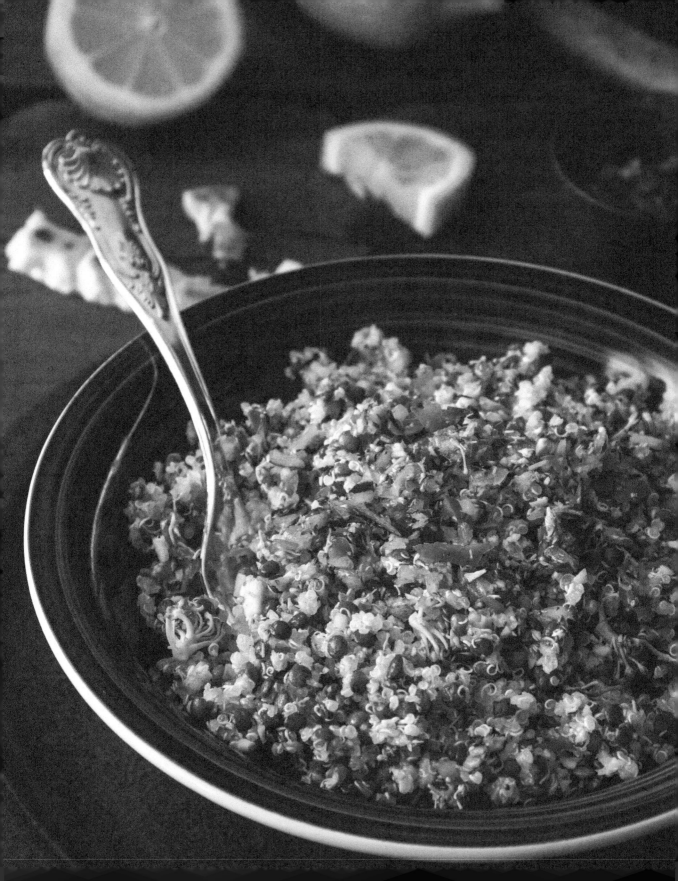

SNACKS and SIDES

4

PUMPKIN and CARROT CRACKERS

MAKES 40 CRACKERS   PREP TIME: 10 MINUTES   COOK TIME: 15 MINUTES

Homemade crackers really don't require a lot of time and effort. Unlike most purchased crackers, this recipe is grain-free—it uses pumpkin seeds as a base. These seeds are a potent source of the mineral zinc, which helps boost the immune system. Say "hello" to your new best anti-inflammatory friend!

1⅓ cups pumpkin seeds

½ cup tightly packed shredded carrot (about 1 carrot)

3 tablespoons chopped fresh dill

2 tablespoons extra-virgin olive oil

¼ teaspoon salt

1   Preheat the oven to 350°F.

2   Line a baking sheet with parchment paper.

3   In a food processor, pulverize the pumpkin seeds into a fine meal.

4   Add the carrot, dill, olive oil, and salt. Pulse for 30 seconds to incorporate all.

5   Transfer the dough to the prepared sheet and pat it out into a rough rectangular shape.

6   Place another sheet of parchment over the dough. Roll the dough to about ⅛ inch thick.

7   Gently score the crackers with a knife or pizza cutter.

8   Place the sheet in the preheated oven and bake for 15 minutes, or until lightly golden.

9   Cool the crackers, separate them, and store in a sealed container.

COOKING TIP: *Roll the crackers out as uniformly thin as you can to ensure even cooking. If some crackers brown too quickly, remove them from the oven before they burn and leave the rest of the batch to bake.*

PER SERVING (4 crackers) Calories: 131; Total Fat: 12g; Total Carbohydrates: 4g; Sugar: 0g; Fiber: 1g; Protein: 5g; Sodium: 67mg

EASY VEGETABLE CRACKERS

MAKES 20 TO 24   PREP TIME: 10 MINUTES   COOK TIME: 1 HOUR 30 MINUTES

CORN FREE
DAIRY FREE
EGG FREE
GLUTEN FREE
NIGHTSHADE FREE
NUT FREE
SOY FREE
PALEO
VEGAN

You'll love it! This recipe has none of the hassle of rolling out crackers. All you do is spread the dough in one large piece that you break up later. These crackers dry instead of roast in the oven. As every oven is unique and special (like you!), it can take anywhere from 1 to 2 hours until the crackers are completely dry. Don't forget about them! Set a kitchen timer or your phone to remind you to check.

½ small green cabbage head, chopped

1 zucchini, grated

1 carrot, grated

¾ cup ground flaxseed

¼ cup water, plus additional as needed

2 tablespoons extra-virgin olive oil

¾ teaspoon salt

1   Preheat the oven to 275°F.

2   Line a baking sheet with parchment paper.

3   In a food processor, combine the cabbage, zucchini, carrot, flaxseed, water, olive oil, and salt. Process until mostly smooth. If the mixture seems dry, add more water, 1 tablespoon at a time.

4   With a spatula, spread the cracker mixture evenly over the prepared sheet.

5   Place the sheet in the preheated oven and bake for 1½ hours, checking every 30 minutes to see how the crackers are drying. They're done when they are completely dry and crispy.

6   Remove from the oven and cool completely.

7   Break into pieces and store in a sealed container.

STORAGE TIP: *To keep crackers and other baked goods fresh, toss a small desiccant packet (the kind often found in vitamin supplement bottles) into the storage container. This absorbs moisture so you don't end up with soggy crackers or muffins.*

PER SERVING (4 crackers) Calories: 163; Total Fat: 11g; Total Carbohydrates: 11g; Sugar: 3g; Fiber: 7g; Protein: 5g; Sodium: 377mg

NO-BAKE CHOCOLATE CHIP GRANOLA BARS

MAKES 10 BARS   PREP TIME: 10 MINUTES   COOK TIME: 5 MINUTES

CORN FREE
DAIRY FREE
EGG FREE
GLUTEN FREE
NIGHTSHADE FREE
SOY FREE
PALEO
VEGAN

These dense little granola bars pack a nutritional punch of protein, fiber, healthy fats, and minerals. You don't need a large bar to feel satisfied—a small square is a perfect mid-morning snack or after-noon pick-me-up.

1½ cups pecans

⅓ cup unsweetened
shredded coconut flakes

¼ cup dairy-free
chocolate chips

⅓ cup sunflower seed butter

⅓ cup maple syrup,
or raw honey

3 tablespoons coconut oil

1   Line a loaf pan with parchment paper.

2   In a food processor, grind the pecans into a coarse flour. Transfer to a medium bowl.

3   Add the coconut flakes and chocolate chips.

4   In a small pot set over low heat, gently melt the sunflower seed butter, maple syrup, and coconut oil together until smooth, about 5 minutes.

5   Pour the wet mixture over the dry ingredients. Stir well to ensure everything is incorporated.

6   Press the granola mixture into the prepared pan.

7   Refrigerate for 2 hours, and then slice into bars. Cover and keep refrigerated until ready to serve.

SUBSTITUTION TIP: *For those with nut allergies, substitute sunflower seeds or pumpkin seeds, or a mix, for the pecans.*

PER SERVING Calories: 305; Total Fat: 25g; Total Carbohydrates: 21g; Sugar: 14g; Fiber: 4g; Protein: 4g; Sodium: 60mg

BAKED ZUCCHINI CHIPS

SERVES 6   PREP TIME: 15 MINUTES   COOK TIME: 2 HOURS

CORN FREE
DAIRY FREE
EGG FREE
GLUTEN FREE
NIGHTSHADE FREE
NUT FREE
SOY FREE
PALEO
VEGAN

Chips don't have to be greasy, inflammatory fat bombs when you make them with nutrient-rich vegetables. Once you master this technique (it's easy), experiment with other vegetables, like yams, butternut squash, beets, parsnips, and carrots.

2 medium zucchini, sliced thin with a mandoline or sharp knife

2 tablespoons extra-virgin olive oil

1½ teaspoons dried basil

1½ teaspoons dried oregano

1½ teaspoons dried rosemary

½ teaspoon salt

1   Preheat the oven to its lowest setting, usually 175°F to 200°F.

2   Line two baking sheets with parchment paper.

3   In a large bowl, toss the zucchini with the olive oil.

4   In a small bowl, stir together the basil, oregano, rosemary, and salt. Pour the herbs over the zucchini. With your hands, mix everything to ensure the zucchini is evenly coated.

5   Place the zucchini in a single layer on the prepared sheets. They can be close together.

6   Place the sheets in the preheated oven and bake for about 2 hours, or until dry and crispy. Baking time will depend on your oven's lowest temperature, and how thin you cut the zucchini.

7   Cool completely. Store in a sealed container.

COOKING TIP: *Any spice you like works well in this recipe! Experiment and have fun.*

PER SERVING Calories: 53; Total Fat: 5g; Total Carbohydrates: 3g; Sugar: 1g; Fiber: 1g; Protein: 1g; Sodium: 201mg

BUTTERNUT SQUASH FRIES

SERVES 4   PREP TIME: 20 MINUTES   COOK TIME: 40 TO 45 MINUTES

CORN FREE
DAIRY FREE
EGG FREE
GLUTEN FREE
NIGHTSHADE FREE
NUT FREE
SOY FREE
PALEO
VEGAN

When you get right down to it, any vegetable can be turned into French fries—so there is no need to miss potatoes. Carrots, butternut squash, parsnips, sweet potatoes, and celery root can all be transformed into French fry-like bites. Root vegetables work especially well as they have that sweet, creamy, carby texture of potatoes. I've also used zucchini and eggplant as a fry substitute. Butternut squash requires a bit of extra work to peel and seed, but the effort is rewarded when you take that first bite.

1 large butternut squash, peeled, seeded, and cut into fry-size pieces, about 3 inches long and ½ inch thick

2 tablespoons coconut oil

¾ teaspoon salt

3 fresh rosemary sprigs, stemmed and chopped (about 1½ tablespoons)

1   Preheat the oven to 375°F.

2   Line a large baking sheet with parchment paper or aluminum foil.

3   In a large bowl, toss the squash pieces with the coconut oil and salt. Scatter the butternut squash over the prepared sheet.

4   Place the sheet in the preheated oven and bake for 20 minutes. Flip the fries over.

5   Continue baking for 10 minutes more.

6   Sprinkle the fries with the rosemary. Bake for 10 to 15 minutes more, or until the fries are golden on the outside.

7   Serve hot.

PREPARATION TIP: *Depending on your preference, cut the squash into whatever shape you like, from matchsticks to wedges. Experiment and see what size you enjoy the most. Depending on the size of the cut, you may need to adjust the time in the oven.*

PER SERVING Calories: 192; Total Fat: 7g; Total Carbohydrates: 34g; Sugar: 6g; Fiber: 7g; Protein: 3g; Sodium: 450mg

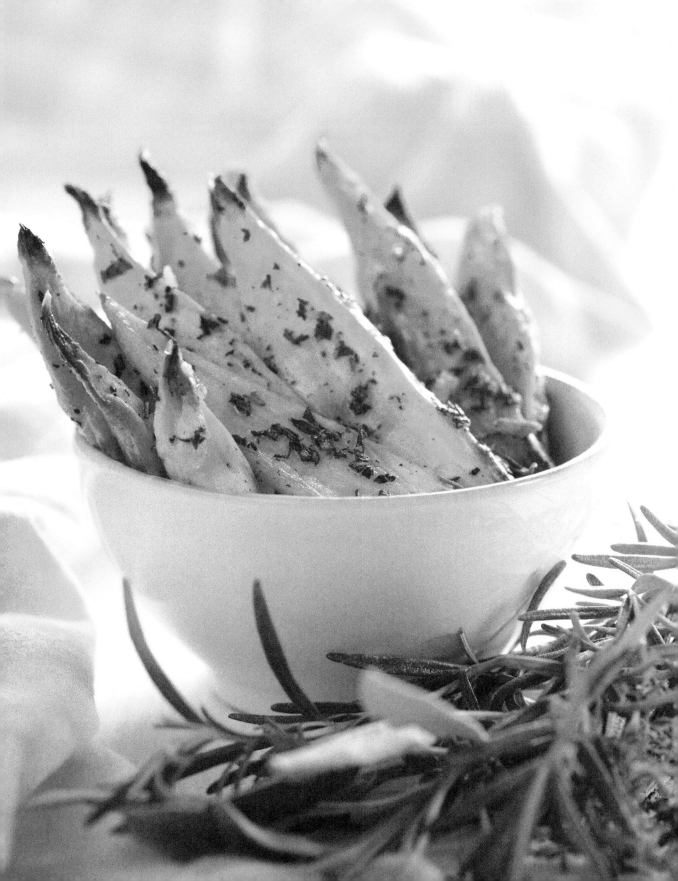

HOMEMADE TRAIL MIX

SERVES 12 TO 14   PREP TIME: 5 MINUTES   COOK TIME: 0 MINUTES

CORN FREE
DAIRY FREE
EGG FREE
GLUTEN FREE
NIGHTSHADE FREE
NUT FREE
SOY FREE
PALEO
VEGAN

This easy, portable snack can be eaten on its own or used as a topping for nondairy yogurt, oatmeal, or fruit for an extra boost of protein and healthy fat. If you want to add the rich flavor of chocolate chips without the added processed sugar, throw in some cacao nibs. When they're eaten with a variety of nuts, seeds, and sweet dried fruit, cacao nibs taste just like chocolate chips.

1 cup pumpkin seeds

1 cup sunflower seeds

1 cup large coconut flakes

1 cup raisins

1 cup dried cranberries

½ cup cacao nibs (optional)

1   In a large bowl, stir together the pumpkin seeds, sunflower seeds, coconut, raisins, cranberries, and cacao nibs (if using).

2   Store, covered, in large jars in a cool, dry place, or portion into small containers for a quick grab-and-go option.

INGREDIENT TIP: *Cacao nibs come from whole cacao beans that have been peeled and crumbled. They have a bitter, pure chocolate flavor and are a rich source of antioxidants.*

PER SERVING Calories: 183; Total Fat: 11g; Total Carbohydrates: 19g; Sugar: 12g; Fiber: 3g; Protein: 5g; Sodium: 24mg

ROASTED APRICOTS

SERVES 4   PREP TIME: 10 MINUTES   COOK TIME: 25 TO 30 MINUTES

CORN FREE
DAIRY FREE
EGG FREE
GLUTEN FREE
NIGHTSHADE FREE
NUT FREE
SOY FREE
PALEO
VEGAN

Cold, raw fruit is undoubtedly sweet and delicious. Still, it's sometimes nice to eat fruit roasted, which brings out even more of its natural sweetness. The final product is soft and oozy, but in the best possible way. These roasted apricots are delicious on their own or topped with nuts, seeds, granola, or coconut yogurt.

20 fresh apricots, pitted and quartered

2 tablespoons coconut oil

⅛ teaspoon cardamom (optional)

1   Preheat the oven to 350°F.

2   In an ovenproof dish, toss the apricots with the coconut oil and cardamom (if using).

3   Place the dish in the preheated oven and roast for 25 to 30 minutes, stirring occasionally.

INGREDIENT TIP: *If you have any leftovers, freeze them in ice cube trays and add to smoothies.*

PER SERVING Calories: 142; Total Fat: 8g; Total Carbohydrates: 19g; Sugar: 16g; Fiber: 3g; Protein: 2g; Sodium: 2mg

QUINOA FLATBREAD

SERVES 8 TO 10   PREP TIME: 5 MINUTES   COOK TIME: 25 TO 30 MINUTES

CORN FREE
DAIRY FREE
EGG FREE
GLUTEN FREE
NIGHTSHADE FREE
NUT FREE
SOY FREE
VEGAN

This hearty, nutty flatbread is an outstanding source of protein, fiber, and minerals like magnesium, folate, and zinc. Flatbread is very versatile. It can be paired with a favorite dip, cut into slices for sandwich bread, or used as the best base for flatbread pizza. It is also delicious grilled or stuffed with your favorite veggies.

1½ cups dry quinoa
2¼ cups water

¼ cup extra-virgin olive oil
1 teaspoon salt

1   Preheat the oven to 350°F.

2   Line a 9-by-13-inch baking pan (or a baking sheet with 1-inch sides) with parchment paper.

3   Using a spice grinder or high-speed blender, pulverize the quinoa into a fine meal. Transfer to a medium bowl.

4   Add the water, olive oil, and salt. Whisk well so there are no lumps.

5   Pour the batter into the prepared pan and smooth it. The batter will be quite wet.

6   Place the pan in the preheated oven and bake for 25 to 30 minutes, or until the flatbread is dry and lightly golden on top.

7   Cut into desired sizes and serve.

EQUIPMENT TIP: *If you don't have a large baking dish or pan, divide the batter between two square or round baking pans (this is great when you're making pizza).*

PER SERVING Calories: 171; Total Fat: 8g; Total Carbohydrates: 21g; Sugar: 0g; Fiber: 2g; Protein: 5g; Sodium: 292mg

CRISPY ROASTED CHICKPEAS

SERVES 8   PREP TIME: 5 MINUTES   COOK TIME: 1 HOUR 30 MINUTES

CORN FREE
DAIRY FREE
EGG FREE
GLUTEN FREE
NIGHTSHADE FREE
NUT FREE
SOY FREE
VEGAN

These tasty treats are a great alternative to potato chips! I like to use dried chickpeas, as they're less expensive and I can control how much salt I use to cook them. Also, soaking the chickpeas helps release the complex carbohydrates that cause gas, and dissipates the phytic acid that binds to vitamins and minerals. Snack attack warning: these can be addictive.

1 cup dried chickpeas, soaked in water for 8 hours

2 teaspoons extra-virgin olive oil

1 tablespoon garlic powder, plus additional as needed

1 teaspoon onion powder, plus additional as needed

¾ teaspoon salt, plus additional as needed

1   Drain the chickpeas and rinse well. Place them in a large pot and cover with a few inches of water. Bring to a boil over medium-high heat. Cook for about 45 minutes, or until tender. Drain again.

2   Preheat the oven to 325°F.

3   Line a large baking sheet with aluminum foil.

4   In a large bowl, toss together the chickpeas, olive oil, garlic powder, onion powder, and salt.

5   Taste, and adjust the seasoning if necessary. Remember that the flavors intensify as the chickpeas bake. »

6   Spread the chickpeas onto the prepared sheet. Depending on the size of your sheet, you may need two—don't crowd the chickpeas.

7   Carefully place the sheet(s) in the preheated oven and bake for about 45 minutes, stirring and turning the chickpeas every 15 minutes, or until golden and crunchy. The chickpeas will also crisp as they cool.

INGREDIENT TIP: *One cup of dried chickpeas yields about three cups cooked chickpeas. If you want to skip the cooking step, substitute two (15-ounce), BPA-free cans of chickpeas. Rinse them well to reduce excess sodium.*

PER SERVING Calories: 106; Total Fat: 3g; Total Carbohydrates: 16g; Sugar: 3g; Fiber: 5g; Protein: 5g; Sodium: 223mg

CUMIN-ROASTED CAULIFLOWER

SERVES 6   PREP TIME: 8 MINUTES   COOK TIME: 25 MINUTES

CORN FREE
DAIRY FREE
EGG FREE
GLUTEN FREE
NIGHTSHADE FREE
NUT FREE
SOY FREE
PALEO
VEGAN

Roasting vegetables brings out their sweet flavor and can make virtually any vegetable taste better. Cruciferous vegetables have a strong taste due to their sulfur content—a detoxifying nutrient—but roasting them with spices makes them far more appetizing to picky palates.

2 medium cauliflower heads, broken into florets (about 8 cups)

3 tablespoons melted coconut oil

2 tablespoons ground cumin

1 teaspoon ground coriander

1 teaspoon salt

1   Preheat the oven to 400°F.

2   In a large bowl, combine the cauliflower, coconut oil, cumin, coriander, and salt. Toss to coat.

3   Transfer the florets to a large roasting tray, or two baking sheets.

4   Place the tray in the preheated oven and bake for 25 minutes, or until the cauliflower is tender and beginning to brown on the edges.

COOKING TIP: *The healthy fats in extra-virgin olive oil and omega-3 oils like flaxseed, chia seed, and hemp seed, are very sensitive to heat, light, and air. High-heat cooking can destroy the beneficial nutrients in these oils and create free radicals. Coconut oil and animal fat (ghee, lard, etc.) are more stable for cooking at high temperatures.*

PER SERVING Calories: 114; Total Fat: 7g; Total Carbohydrates: 11g; Sugar: 5g; Fiber: 5g; Protein: 4g; Sodium: 448mg

SMASHED PEAS

SERVES 4   PREP TIME: 10 MINUTES   COOK TIME: 8 TO 10 MINUTES

CORN FREE
DAIRY FREE
EGG FREE
GLUTEN FREE
NIGHTSHADE FREE
NUT FREE
SOY FREE
PALEO
VEGAN

This satisfying, creamy side dish is another option to replace white potatoes. The peas are sweet and creamy and the herbs make certain they aren't the same old "peas and carrots." Similar to other green foods, peas are a rich source of nutrients like B vitamins, antioxidants like vitamins A and C, magnesium, iron, omega-3s, potassium, and fiber. Aren't green foods awesome?

4 cups frozen peas, thawed

¼ cup extra-virgin olive oil

¼ cup fresh mint, chopped

¼ cup fresh dill, chopped

1 teaspoon salt, plus additional as needed

1   Fill a pot with 2 inches of water and insert a steamer basket. Place it over high heat and bring to a boil.

2   Add the peas. Cover and cook for 8 to 10 minutes, or until the peas are bright green and tender. Drain and transfer to a food processor.

3   Add the olive oil, mint, dill, and salt.

4   Process until completely smooth, or pulse a few times and leave some texture.

5   Taste, and adjust the seasoning if necessary.

EQUIPMENT TIP: *If you don't have a food processor (or don't feel like washing another appliance), use a potato masher or a fork to smash the peas.*

PER SERVING Calories: 243; Total Fat: 13g; Total Carbohydrates: 25g; Sugar: 7g; Fiber: 10g; Protein: 9g; Sodium: 705mg

HERB-STUFFED STEAMED RICE

SERVES 6 TO 8   PREP TIME: 10 MINUTES   COOK TIME: 45 MINUTES

CORN FREE
DAIRY FREE
EGG FREE
GLUTEN FREE
NIGHTSHADE FREE
NUT FREE
SOY FREE
VEGAN

This pleasantly fragrant side dish is perfect for fresh herb lovers. You read right—there are three bunches of herbs in this, but when finely minced the volume decreases considerably. If you like herbs, but not quite this much, halve the amounts or choose small bunches.

2 cups short-grain brown rice

4 cups water

1½ teaspoons salt

1 bunch fresh basil, washed, stemmed, and finely chopped

1 bunch fresh dill, washed, stemmed, and finely chopped

1 bunch parsley, washed, stemmed, and finely chopped

1   In a fine-mesh strainer, rinse the rice well and transfer to a large pot set over medium-high heat. Add the water and salt. Bring to a boil. Cover and simmer for 30 minutes.

2   Add the herbs to the pot and stir well.

3   Cook for 15 minutes more, or until the rice is tender and chewy.

INGREDIENT TIP: *You can use any type of brown rice here—long grain, basmati, jasmine—choose the shape and style you prefer!*

PER SERVING Calories: 241; Total Fat: 2g; Total Carbohydrates: 54g; Sugar: 1g; Fiber: 5g; Protein: 5g; Sodium: 595mg

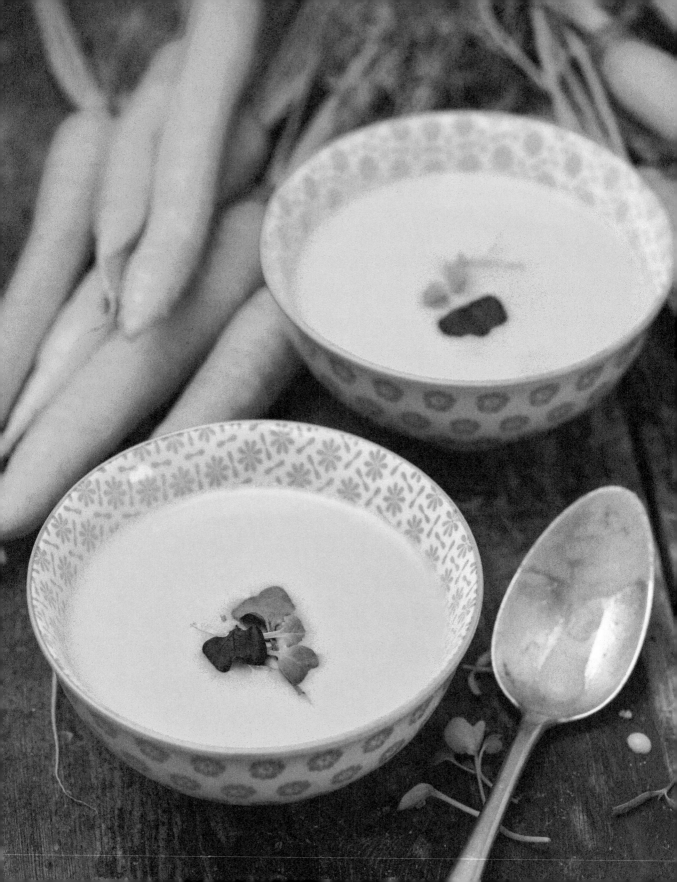

SOUPS and SALADS

5

GLUTEN-FREE RAMEN "TO GO"

SERVES 1   PREP TIME: 10 MINUTES   COOK TIME: 5 MINUTES

CORN FREE
DAIRY FREE
EGG FREE
GLUTEN FREE
NIGHTSHADE FREE
NUT FREE
SOY FREE
VEGAN

No need for cup-a-soup or instant noodles when you've got this recipe in your repertoire—an easy, portable grab-and-go lunch made with fresh ingredients. This recipe is designed to fit in a 1 pint mason jar. If you're really hungry, stuff in more vegetables and use a bigger container.

½ cup cooked soba noodles, or soaked and drained rice noodles

½ cup grated carrot

1 large kale leaf, thoroughly washed and finely chopped

1 tablespoon tahini

1 teaspoon dried vegetable broth powder

⅛ teaspoon salt

Boiling water, to cover

1   In a 1 pint mason jar, layer the soba noodles, carrot, kale, tahini, broth powder, and salt. Seal the jar. Refrigerate or pack in your lunchbox.

2   When you're ready to eat, bring a kettle of water to a boil. Fill the jar with enough water to cover the vegetables. Reseal the lid and steep the soup for 4 to 5 minutes.

3   Stir well to incorporate the seasoning, and enjoy.

INGREDIENT TIP: *Make this recipe Paleo by using spiralized zucchini noodles instead of buckwheat or rice noodles.*

PER SERVING Calories: 206; Total Fat: 8g; Total Carbohydrates: 29g; Sugar: 3g; Fiber: 4g; Protein: 8g; Sodium: 818mg

SLOW-COOKER VEGAN SPLIT PEA SOUP

SERVES 8   PREP TIME: 10 MINUTES   COOK TIME: 4 TO 8 HOURS

CORN FREE
DAIRY FREE
EGG FREE
GLUTEN FREE
NIGHTSHADE FREE
NUT FREE
SOY FREE
VEGAN

When packed with filling ingredients, any soup can become a complete meal. This thick, hearty, and warming split pea soup will satisfy all the hungry appetites at the table. Depending on your preference, blend the soup completely or blend only half, which will leave some textured mouthfuls.

6½ cups water

2½ cups green or yellow split peas, rinsed well

2 small sweet potatoes, cut into ½-inch dice

1 tablespoon dried thyme

1½ teaspoons salt, plus additional as needed

1   In a slow cooker, combine the water, split peas, sweet potatoes, thyme, and salt.

2   Cover and cook on low for 8 hours, or on high for 4 hours.

3   Using an immersion blender or in a regular blender, blend half (or all) of the soup, working in batches as needed and taking care with the hot liquid.

4   Taste and adjust the seasoning, if necessary.

COOKING TIP: *No slow cooker? Simmer this soup on the stove for 1½ to 2 hours. You may need to add more liquid as it cooks.*

NOTE *that the Week One Plan calls for leftovers; double the quantities so you have enough for later in the week.*

PER SERVING Calories: 51; Total Fat: 0g; Total Carbohydrates: 12g; Sugar: 0g; Fiber: 2g; Protein: 1g; Sodium: 448mg

CARROT-GINGER SOUP

SERVES 6 TO 8   PREP TIME: 10 MINUTES   COOK TIME: 30 MINUTES

This creamy soup combines two powerful anti-inflammatory ingredients in one comforting bowl. Depending on your tolerance for ginger, add more or less than what is called for here.

1 large onion, peeled and roughly chopped

4½ cups plus 2 tablespoons water, divided

8 carrots, peeled and roughly chopped (see Tip)

1½-inch piece fresh ginger, sliced thin (see Tip)

1¼ teaspoons salt

2 cups coconut milk

1   In a large pot set over medium heat, sauté the onion in 2 tablespoons of water for about 5 minutes, or until soft.

2   Add the carrots, the remaining 4½ cups of water, the ginger, and salt. Bring to a boil. Reduce the heat to low and cover the pot. Simmer for 20 minutes.

3   Stir in the coconut milk and let it heat for 4 to 5 minutes.

4   In a blender, blend the soup until creamy, working in batches if necessary and taking care with the hot liquid.

PREPARATION TIP: *You don't have to peel the carrots or ginger if they're organic—leave the skin on and wash them well.*

NOTE *that the Week Three Plan calls for leftovers; double the quantities so you have enough for later in the week.*

PER SERVING Calories: 228; Total Fat: 19g; Total Carbohydrates: 15g; Sugar: 8g; Fiber: 4g; Protein: 3g; Sodium: 554mg

CREAM OF BROCCOLI SOUP

SERVES 6   PREP TIME: 12 MINUTES   COOK TIME: 25 MINUTES

CORN FREE
DAIRY FREE
EGG FREE
GLUTEN FREE
NIGHTSHADE FREE
SOY FREE
PALEO
VEGAN

You don't need dairy to enjoy an ultra-creamy soup. This recipe uses soaked cashews instead to provide a rich, buttery texture. Don't toss the broccoli stalks—chop them and cook them, too. Since everything is blended in the end, you don't even have to peel the tough outer stalk; it will soften during cooking.

1 onion, finely chopped

4 garlic cloves, finely chopped

5 cups plus 2 tablespoons water, divided

1½ teaspoons salt, plus additional as needed

4 broccoli heads with stalks, heads cut into florets and stalks roughly chopped

1 cup cashews, soaked in water for at least 4 hours

1   In a large pot set over medium heat, sauté the onion and garlic in 2 tablespoons of water for about 5 minutes, or until soft.

2   Add the remaining 5 cups of water, the salt, and the broccoli. Bring to a boil. Cover and reduce the heat to low. Simmer for 20 minutes.

3   Drain and rinse the cashews. Transfer them to a blender.

4   Add the soup to the blender. Blend until smooth, working in batches if necessary, and taking care with the hot liquid. Taste, and adjust the seasoning if necessary.

SUBSTITUTION TIP: *If you are allergic to nuts, use one cup of soaked sun-flower seeds instead.*

NOTE *that the Week Two Plan calls for leftovers; double the quantities so you have enough for later in the week.*

PER SERVING Calories: 224; Total Fat: 11g; Total Carbohydrates: 26g; Sugar: 6g; Fiber: 7g; Protein: 11g; Sodium: 85mg

CLASSIC BUTTERNUT SQUASH SOUP

SERVES 6   PREP TIME: 20 MINUTES   COOK TIME: 30 MINUTES

CORN FREE
DAIRY FREE
EGG FREE
GLUTEN FREE
NIGHTSHADE FREE
NUT FREE
SOY FREE
PALEO
VEGAN

Butternut squash can be unwieldy to handle and it does take some time to chop, but the results are worth it. The creamy, potato-like texture is packed with nutrients like vitamin A and *cucurbitacins*, highly anti-inflammatory phytochemicals. Dicing butternut squash is a perfect "do ahead" task to take on during the weekend, and the process is much easier with a good, sharp knife. Refrigerate the cubes for 5 days, or freeze for several months. I like to cut up a couple at a time and stash cubes in the freezer for later.

1 onion, roughly chopped

4½ cups plus 2 tablespoons water, divided

1 large butternut squash, washed, peeled, ends trimmed, halved, seeded, and cut into ½-inch chunks

2 celery stalks, roughly chopped

3 carrots, peeled and roughly chopped

1 teaspoon salt, plus additional as needed

1   In a large pot set over medium heat, sauté the onion in 2 tablespoons of water for about 5 minutes, or until soft.

2   Add the squash, celery, carrot, and salt. Bring to a boil.

3   Reduce the heat to low, Cover and simmer for 25 minutes.

4   In a blender, purée the soup until smooth, working in batches if necessary and taking care with the hot liquid. Taste, and adjust the seasoning if necessary.

SUBSTITUTION TIP: *Substitute any variety of winter squash you like. This soup is also delicious made with sweet potatoes! To save some prep time, purchase precut squash at the grocery store.*

NOTE *that the Week Two Plan calls for leftovers from the end of Week One; double the quantities so you have enough for the next week.*

PER SERVING Calories: 104; Total Fat: 0g; Total Carbohydrates: 27g; Sugar: 6g; Fiber: 5g; Protein: 2g; Sodium: 417mg

THAI SWEET POTATO SOUP

SERVES 4 TO 6   PREP TIME: 10 MINUTES   COOK TIME: 20 TO 25 MINUTES

CORN FREE
DAIRY FREE
EGG FREE
GLUTEN FREE
NIGHTSHADE FREE
SOY FREE
PALEO
VEGAN

This soup is perfect for warming you on those wintry days when you begin to feel the chill in your fingers, nose, and toes. This is a pared-down version of Thai soup; if you have extra prep time and ingredients in your refrigerator, toss in some onions and garlic, serve with rice noodles and spinach, or garnish with more lime wedges, chopped nuts, and scallions. Better yet, create a "Thai Soup Bar" where everyone can choose their own adventure!

3 large sweet potatoes, cubed

2 cups water

1 (14-ounce) can coconut milk

½-inch piece fresh ginger, sliced

½ cup almond butter

Zest of 1 lime

Juice of 1 lime

1 teaspoon salt, plus additional as needed

1   In a large pot set over high heat, combine the sweet potatoes, water, coconut milk, and ginger. Bring to a boil. Reduce the heat to low and cover.

2   Simmer for 20 to 25 minutes, or until the potatoes are tender. Transfer the potatoes, ginger, and cooking liquid to a blender.

3   Add the almond butter, lime zest, lime juice, and salt.

4   Blend until smooth.

5   Taste, and adjust the seasoning if necessary.

INGREDIENT TIP: *If you like heat and don't mind nightshades, add a few Thai red chiles—the teeny, slender, bright red chiles are often available at grocery stores.*

PER SERVING Calories: 653; Total Fat: 42g; Total Carbohydrates: 64g; Sugar: 4g; Fiber: 11g; Protein: 12g; Sodium: 614mg

CHICKPEA and KALE SALAD

SERVES 4   PREP TIME: 10 MINUTES   COOK TIME: 20 MINUTES

CORN FREE
DAIRY FREE
EGG FREE
GLUTEN FREE
NUT FREE
SOY FREE
VEGAN

I know what you're thinking: raw kale is not for me. Hold that thought. The secret to eating and enjoying kale raw is giving it a good massage with lemon juice and salt first. This helps wilt and break down the greens, so they're more palatable and easier to digest. Once you give your kale some love, it will love you right back with its wonderful taste and healthy nutrients.

1 large bunch kale, thoroughly washed, stemmed, and cut into thin strips

2 teaspoons freshly squeezed lemon juice

2 tablespoons extra-virgin olive oil, divided

¾ teaspoon salt, divided

2 cups cooked chickpeas (about 1 [14-oz] can)

1 teaspoon sweet paprika

1 avocado, chopped (optional)

1   In a large bowl, combine the kale, lemon juice, 1 tablespoon of olive oil, and ¼ teaspoon of salt.

2   With your hands, massage the kale for 5 minutes, or until it starts to wilt and becomes bright green and shiny.

3   To a skillet set over medium-low heat, add the remaining 1 tablespoon of olive oil.

4   Stir in the chickpeas, paprika, and remaining ½ teaspoon of salt. Cook for about 15 minutes, or until warm. The chickpeas might start to crisp in spots.

5   Pour the chickpeas over the kale. Toss well. Add the avocado (if using).

6   Serve immediately.

SUBSTITUTION TIP: *If you don't want to use paprika, you can substitute many other herbs and spices. Dried basil, oregano, dill, parsley, garlic or onion powder, cumin, or turmeric also work well. You can also omit the herbs and just use salt.*

PER SERVING Calories: 359; Total Fat: 20g; Total Carbohydrates: 35g; Sugar: 1g; Fiber: 10g; Protein: 13g; Sodium: 497mg

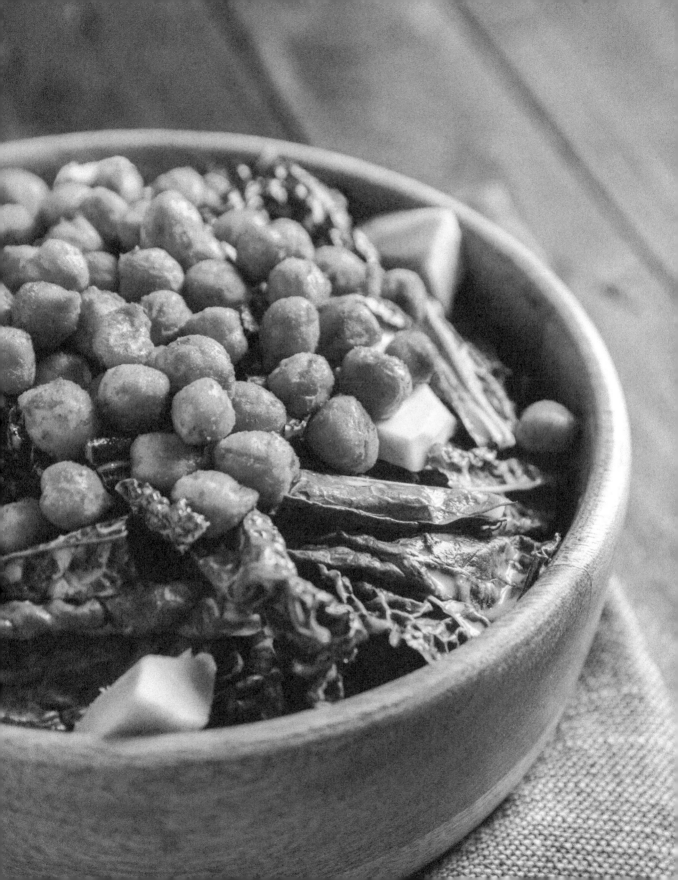

GLORIOUS CREAMED GREENS SOUP

SERVES 4 TO 6   PREP TIME: 10 MINUTES   COOK TIME: 15 MINUTES

Eating dark leafy greens is like consuming a natural multivitamin. They are packed with so many anti-inflammatory nutrients, plus they are an amazing source of fiber and micro-minerals. It might seem like a lot of greens in this recipe, but they shrink a *lot* after cooking. The trick is to add the greens to the pot a little at a time.

3 cups water

2 cups coconut milk

1½ teaspoons salt, plus additional as needed

4 cups tightly packed kale, thoroughly washed, stemmed, and roughly chopped

4 cups tightly packed spinach, stemmed and roughly chopped

4 cups tightly packed collard greens, stemmed and roughly chopped

1 bunch fresh parsley, stemmed and roughly chopped

1   In a large pot set over high heat, bring the water, coconut milk, and salt to a boil. Reduce the heat to low.

2   Add the kale, spinach, and collard greens 1 cup at a time, letting them wilt before adding the next cup. Continue until all the greens have been added to the pot.

3   Simmer for 8 to 10 minutes.

4   In a blender, blend the soup until smooth, working in batches if necessary and taking care with the hot liquid.

5   Taste, and adjust the seasoning (if necessary) before serving.

SUBSTITUTION TIP: *Any dark leafy green will work in this soup. Pick the ones you love, or use what you have in the refrigerator.*

NOTE *that the Week Three Plan calls for leftovers; double the quantities so you have enough later in the week.*

PER SERVING Calories: 334; Total Fat: 29g; Total Carbohydrates: 18g; Sugar: 4g; Fiber: 6g; Protein: 7g; Sodium: 959mg

BASIC CHICKEN BROTH (BONE BROTH)

SERVES 6 TO 8 PREP TIME: 10 MINUTES COOK TIME: 8 TO 24 HOURS

CORN FREE
DAIRY FREE
EGG FREE
GLUTEN FREE
NIGHTSHADE FREE
NUT FREE
SOY FREE
PALEO
VEGAN

Bone broth is an incredibly nourishing food. Made with organic animal bones full of anti-inflammatory nutrients, it supports digestion, aids joint health, and helps build connective tissues. Cooking the bones for long periods of time means all of these vital nutrients leach into the water. I visit my local butcher for a few pounds of chicken bones, or use the leftover carcass from a roasted chicken dinner. The apple cider vinegar further helps to pull the nutrients out of the bones, but it's completely optional if you don't have it in your pantry.

2 pounds organic chicken bones, or 1 leftover organic chicken carcass

1 small onion, quartered, skin on

1-inch piece fresh ginger, roughly chopped

1 small bunch fresh fennel, roughly chopped

1 small bunch fresh parsley, roughly chopped

10 to 12 cups cold water

1 tablespoon apple cider vinegar (optional)

1 In a slow cooker, combine the chicken bones, onion, ginger, fennel, parsley, water, and cider vinegar (if using). The amount of water needed will depend on the size of your cooker. Cover everything by 1 to 2 inches.

2 Cover and cook on low for a minimum of 8 hours.

3 Strain the broth, discarding the vegetables and bones. Cover and refrigerate until needed.

COOKING TIP: *This broth can also be made on the stove top. Simmer for 4 to 6 hours over low heat. If you want to keep this even more basic and cut down on prep work, add just the bones and water to the slow cooker. You'll still get all the nutrients from the bones; you just won't get the extra anti-inflammatory boost from the onion and herbs.*

PER SERVING Calories: 86; Total Fat: 2g; Total Carbohydrates: 8g; Sugar: 4g; Fiber: 0g; Protein: 6g; Sodium: 279mg

CREAMY CABBAGE SLAW

SERVES 6   PREP TIME: 20 MINUTES   COOK TIME: 0 MINUTES

CORN FREE
DAIRY FREE
EGG FREE
GLUTEN FREE
NIGHTSHADE FREE
SOY FREE
PALEO
VEGAN

Commercial coleslaws are usually sopping with mayonnaise. This alternative keeps the richness without the eggs, which can cause digestive or allergic reactions in some people. The longer you marinate this slaw, the more it will grab onto the flavors. I recommend making this the day before serving it. The extra marinating time also helps break down the cabbage, making it easier to digest.

1 large head green or red cabbage, sliced thin

2 carrots, grated

1 cup cashews, soaked in water for at least 4 hours

¼ cup freshly squeezed lemon juice

½ to ¾ cup water

¾ teaspoon salt

1   In a large bowl, combine the cabbage and carrots.

2   Drain and rinse the cashews.

3   In a blender, process the cashews with the lemon juice, ½ cup of water, and the salt until smooth and creamy. If the dressing is too thick, add more water, 1 tablespoon at a time.

4   Pour the sauce over the vegetables and mix well. Refrigerate for at least 1 hour before serving to give the vegetables time to marinate.

SUBSTITUTION TIP: *If nut allergies are an issue, substitute soaked sunflower seeds or sesame seeds.*

PER SERVING Calories: 208; Total Fat: 11g; Total Carbohydrates: 25g; Sugar: 4g; Fiber: 8g; Protein: 7g; Sodium: 394mg

CARROT and RAISIN SALAD

SERVES 6   PREP TIME: 12 MINUTES   COOK TIME: 0 MINUTES

CORN FREE
DAIRY FREE
EGG FREE
GLUTEN FREE
NIGHTSHADE FREE
NUT FREE
SOY FREE
PALEO
VEGAN

This simple dish offers a pleasing mix of tastes, textures, and flavors. You get sweetness from the carrots and raisins, the crunchy snap of sunflower seeds, and a bit of lemony tang. If you're making this ahead of time, don't add the seeds until right before serving, as they'll become soggy.

4 cups shredded carrots

1 cup raisins, chopped

¾ cup sunflower seeds

¼ cup maple syrup, plus additional as needed

¼ cup freshly squeezed lemon juice, plus additional as needed

1   In a large bowl, mix together the carrots, raisins, and sunflower seeds.

2   Stir in the maple syrup and lemon juice.

3   Taste, and add more lemon juice or maple syrup if necessary.

SUBSTITUTION TIP: *If nut allergies are not an issue, use chopped almonds, pecans, or walnuts in place of the sunflower seeds.*

PER SERVING Calories: 173; Total Fat: 3g; Total Carbohydrates: 37g; Sugar: 26g; Fiber: 3g; Protein: 3g; Sodium: 57mg

CHILLED SWEET POTATO SALAD

SERVES 6   PREP TIME: 12 MINUTES   COOK TIME: 20 MINUTES

Have you heard of "prebiotics?" These are carbohydrates that feed the good types of bacteria in the colon. One type of prebiotic is resistant starch, which is drawing plenty of attention lately for its benefit to gut health (remember, a healthy gut equals a healthy immune system). Resistant starch increases the colon's production of *butyrate*, a highly anti-inflammatory short chain fatty acid. What's the moral of the story? Cooked and cooled potatoes are high in resistant starch, but since this diet eliminates white potatoes, sweet potatoes take their place in this delicious salad.

4 sweet potatoes, or yams, cut into ½-inch cubes

2 scallions, finely chopped

½ cup fresh dill, finely chopped

¼ cup extra-virgin olive oil

1½ teaspoons salt

1   Fill a large pot with 3 to 4 inches of water and insert a steamer basket. Bring the water to a boil over high heat.

2   Add the sweet potatoes to the steamer basket. Depending on the size of your basket, you may need to do this in two batches. Cover and steam for 8 to 10 minutes, or until the potatoes are firm and tender, but not mushy. Drain, and rinse under cold water to stop the cooking process.

3   In a large bowl, gently combine the sweet potatoes, scallions, dill, olive oil, and salt.

4   Refrigerate until ready to serve.

COOKING TIP: *Love roasted potatoes? You can use the roasting method in this recipe, too. Toss the sweet potatoes with 2 tablespoons of coconut oil and roast at 400°F for 35 to 40 minutes. Cool and proceed with the rest of the recipe.*

PER SERVING Calories: 241; Total Fat: 9g; Total Carbohydrates: 40g; Sugar: 1g; Fiber: 6g; Protein: 3g; Sodium: 601mg

QUINOA-LENTIL SALAD

SERVES 6   PREP TIME: 20 MINUTES   COOK TIME: 45 MINUTES

Salads don't have to mean just iceberg lettuce, cucumber, and tomatoes. There is a wide variety of ingredients you can use to create a salad that is both hearty and satisfying. I love adding beans and grains to salads for an extra boost of anti-inflammatory protein and fiber. Try it; I think you will, too.

1 cup green, brown, or French green lentils

4 cups water, divided

1 cup quinoa

1 broccoli head, finely chopped

4 carrots, grated

⅓ cup extra-virgin olive oil

1 teaspoon salt, plus additional as needed

1   In a fine-mesh strainer, rinse the lentils. Transfer to a medium pot set over high heat and add 2 cups of water. Bring to a boil. Simmer for 15 to 20 minutes, or until tender. Drain off any excess liquid.

2   In a fine-mesh strainer, rinse the quinoa. Transfer to another medium pot set over high heat and add the remaining 2 cups of water. Bring to a boil. Simmer for 15 minutes, or until all the liquid is absorbed. Remove from the heat and let sit for 10 minutes. Fluff with a fork.

3   In a large bowl, combine the lentils, quinoa, broccoli, and carrots.

4   Stir in the olive oil and salt. Taste and adjust the seasoning, if necessary.

5   Refrigerate for at least 1 hour before serving.

MAKE AHEAD TIP: *Precooking large batches of beans and grains makes weekday meal prep a whole lot easier. Cook the quinoa and lentils on the weekend and refrigerate until needed. The vegetables can also be chopped and grated in advance, so all that's left is assembly when you're ready to eat.*

PER SERVING Calories: 369; Total Fat: 16g; Total Carbohydrates: 44g; Sugar: 3g; Fiber: 14g; Protein: 14g; Sodium: 434mg

SIMPLE SPINACH SALAD

SERVES 4   PREP TIME: 10 MINUTES   COOK TIME: 0 MINUTES

CORN FREE
DAIRY FREE
EGG FREE
GLUTEN FREE
NIGHTSHADE FREE
NUT FREE
SOY FREE
PALEO
VEGAN

Everyone needs (and deserves) a good spinach salad recipe in their repertoire. This versatile salad can be thrown together at the last minute for an extra surge of greens to complement virtually any meal, like Grain-Free Fritters (page 111). Pair this with a simple bowl of soup, your favorite stew, roast chicken, chili, or a sandwich, too.

¼ cup extra-virgin olive oil

¼ cup Dijon mustard

2 tablespoons freshly squeezed lemon juice

1½ tablespoons maple syrup

¼ teaspoon salt, plus additional as needed

6 cups baby spinach leaves

1   In a small jar, combine the olive oil, Dijon mustard, lemon juice, maple syrup, and salt. Cover and shake well to mix.

2   Taste, and adjust the seasoning if necessary.

3   In a large serving bowl, toss together the spinach and dressing.

4   Ingredient Tip: If you have extra vegetables or greens in the refrigerator, add them to this dish. Also, a sprinkle of walnuts or sunflower seeds, some dried fruit like dates or cranberries, or fresh fruit such as figs or raspberries add a nice touch.

PER SERVING Calories: 150; Total Fat: 14g; Total Carbohydrates: 8g; Sugar: 5g; Fiber: 2g; Protein: 2g; Sodium: 362mg

GARLICKY SAUTÉED GREENS

SERVES 4 TO 6   PREP TIME: 10 MINUTES   COOK TIME: 8 TO 10 MINUTES

CORN FREE
DAIRY FREE
EGG FREE
GLUTEN FREE
NIGHTSHADE FREE
NUT FREE
SOY FREE
PALEO
VEGAN

If you love garlic (and who doesn't?), you'll be a huge fan of this dish. If you dare, add even more cloves for an extra pungent, garlicky taste.

1 tablespoon coconut oil

8 garlic cloves, minced

3 cups tightly packed chopped kale, thoroughly washed

3 cups tightly packed chopped Swiss chard

Water, for cooking

½ teaspoon salt

2 tablespoons freshly squeezed lemon juice

1   In a large pan set over medium heat, heat the coconut oil.

2   Add the garlic. Cook for 3 to 4 minutes.

3   Add the kale and Swiss chard, 1 cup at a time, letting the greens wilt before adding the next cup.

4   If the pan gets a little dry, add 1 tablespoon of water at a time, as needed.

5   Stir in the salt and lemon juice.

COOKING TIP: *After mincing garlic cloves, wait about five minutes before cooking them. Why? Chopping garlic stimulates the production of allicin, one of garlic's beneficial anti-inflammatory nutrients. However, if you cook garlic too soon after slicing and dicing, the enzymes that manufacture allicin are destroyed.*

PER SERVING Calories: 70; Total Fat: 4g; Total Carbohydrates: 8g; Sugar: 1g; Fiber: 1g; Protein: 2g; Sodium: 373mg

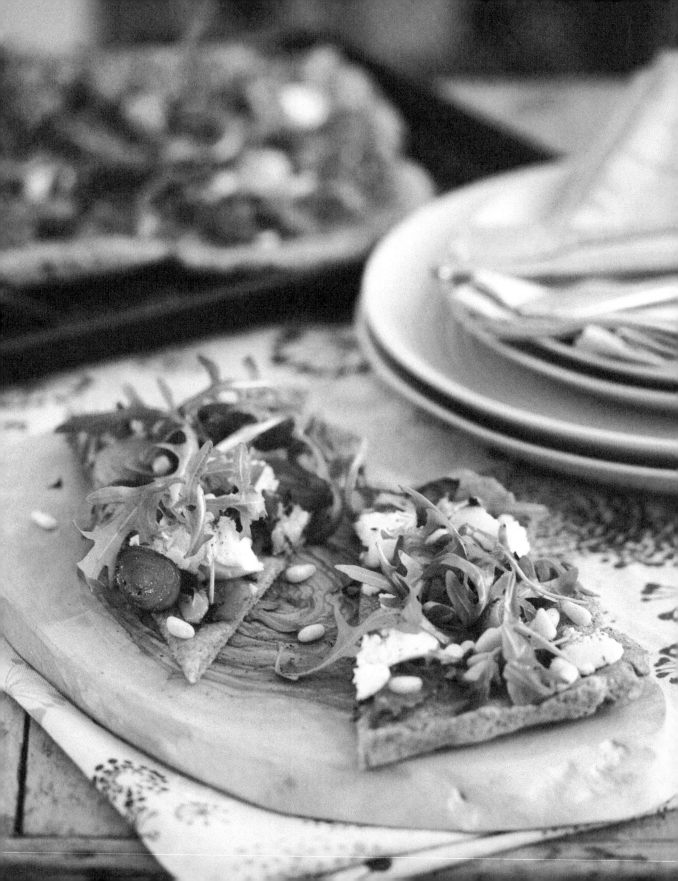

VEGETARIAN DISHES

6

ROOT VEGETABLE LOAF

SERVES 6 TO 8   PREP TIME: 20 MINUTES   COOK TIME: 55 MINUTES TO 1 HOUR

CORN FREE
DAIRY FREE
EGG FREE
GLUTEN FREE
NIGHTSHADE FREE
NUT FREE
SOY FREE
VEGAN

Vegetable loaves can be incredibly warm, satisfying, and comforting—especially on a brisk autumn day. This simple recipe comes together even faster if you use a food processor to grate the vegetables, but a little elbow grease and a box grater work just fine. It also freezes well, so the loaf can be made in advance.

1 onion, finely chopped

2 tablespoons water

2 cups grated carrots

1½ cups grated sweet potatoes

1½ cups gluten-free rolled oats

¾ cup butternut squash purée

1 teaspoon salt

1   Preheat the oven to 350°F.

2   Line a loaf pan with parchment paper.

3   In a large pot set over medium heat, sauté the onion in the water for about 5 minutes, or until soft.

4   Add the carrots and sweet potatoes. Cook for 2 minutes. Remove the pot from the heat.

5   Stir in the oats, butternut squash purée, and salt. Mix well.

6   Transfer the mixture to the prepared loaf pan, pressing down evenly.

7   Place the pan in the preheated oven and bake for 50 to 55 minutes, uncovered, or until the loaf is firm and golden.

8   Cool for 10 minutes before slicing.

INGREDIENT TIP: *Butternut squash purée is easy to make! Steam butternut squash cubes until tender (about 7 minutes) and purée in a food processor or blender. Store the cooked purée in jars in the freezer, or freeze them in ice cube trays (I like to do both!).*

PREPARATION TIP: *You don't have to peel the sweet potatoes if they're organic—leave the skin on and save yourself the extra step!*

PER SERVING Calories: 169; Total Fat: 2g; Total Carbohydrates: 34g; Sugar: 3g; Fiber: 6g; Protein: 5g; Sodium: 442mg

BAKED FALAFEL

SERVES 6 TO 8   PREP TIME: 15 MINUTES   COOK TIME: 30 MINUTES

CORN FREE
DAIRY FREE
EGG FREE
GLUTEN FREE
NIGHTSHADE FREE
NUT FREE
SOY FREE
VEGAN

Falafel is traditionally deep-fried—usually in omega-6 oils at extremely high temperatures, which can definitely contribute to inflammation. This recipe is baked, creating a much healthier and easier option because the cooking is hands off. It's a win-win!

3 cups cooked chickpeas

⅓ cup tahini

1 tablespoon ground cumin

4 garlic cloves

½ teaspoon salt

1 small bunch fresh basil, stemmed and torn into pieces

Water, for thinning

1   Preheat the oven to 350°F.

2   Line a baking sheet with parchment paper.

3   In a food processor, combine the chickpeas, tahini, cumin, garlic, and salt. Process until mostly smooth.

4   Add the basil. Pulse until incorporated.

5   If necessary, add 1 or 2 tablespoons of water to help the ingredients form a ball, being careful not to add too much. The mixture should *not* be wet and pasty.

6   Measure 2 tablespoons of dough and roll it into a ball. Place it on the baking sheet. With the bottom of a glass or your hand, press the ball into a patty about 1 inch thick. Repeat with the remaining chickpea mixture; it should yield about 24 patties.

7   Place the patties in the preheated oven and bake for 30 minutes. The falafels will be quite soft when straight out of the oven, but they firm as they cool.

EQUIPMENT TIP: *A spring-loaded ice cream scoop is an incredibly handy kitchen tool. It's great for scooping ice cream, of course, but it also creates uniform falafels, burger patties, muffins, and cookies. This helps food cook evenly.*

PER SERVING Calories: 242; Total Fat: 12g; Total Carbohydrates: 24g; Sugar: 1g; Fiber: 7g; Protein: 12g; Sodium: 225mg

YAM-BEAN BURGERS

SERVES 4 TO 6   PREP TIME: 15 MINUTES   COOK TIME: 35 MINUTES

CORN FREE
DAIRY FREE
EGG FREE
GLUTEN FREE
NIGHTSHADE FREE
NUT FREE
SOY FREE
VEGAN

Recipes like this are easier to assemble when you've prepped ahead of time. If you cook the beans and yam purée in advance (say, over the weekend), then suddenly homemade yam-bean burgers become a breeze to make and cook, and a treat to eat.

1 cup gluten-free rolled oats

3 cups cooked navy beans (1½ cups dried)

2 cups yam/sweet potato purée (about 2 yams/sweet potatoes, steamed and mashed)

½ cup sunflower seed butter, or tahini

1 tablespoon grated fresh ginger

½ teaspoon salt

1 In a food processor, pulse the oats a few times until a rough meal forms.

2 Add the beans, yam purée, sunflower seed butter, ginger, and salt. Blend until well mixed. You can make this completely smooth, or leave slightly chunky.

3 Refrigerate the mixture for 30 minutes to firm.

4 Preheat the oven to 350°F.

5 Line a baking sheet with parchment paper or Silpat.

6 Using a ⅓-cup or ½-cup measure, scoop the mixture onto the prepared sheet. (The scoop size depends on how large you want the burgers to be.) Gently pat the mixture down so the patties are 1 inch thick. Makes about 12 patties.

7 Place the sheet in the preheated oven and bake for 35 minutes. Flip the burgers halfway through the cooking time.

MAKE AHEAD TIP: *These burgers freeze well. Shape the patties, place them on the baking sheet, and pop the sheet straight into the freezer. Once the burgers are frozen, stack them in a container with a piece of parchment paper between each. Defrost for 15 minutes before baking.*

PER SERVING Calories: 581; Total Fat: 19g; Total Carbohydrates: 81g; Sugar: 6g; Fiber: 26g; Protein: 27g; Sodium: 355mg

BLACK BEAN CHILI

SERVES 6   PREP TIME: 10 MINUTES   COOK TIME: 1 HOUR

CORN FREE
DAIRY FREE
EGG FREE
GLUTEN FREE
NUT FREE
SOY FREE
VEGAN

Fruits and vegetables are "go tos" for antioxidants, but black beans contain high amounts of antioxidant-rich nutrients called *anthocyanins*, which are responsible for their bright, almost purplish color. Another classic chili option, kidney beans, can also be used in this recipe.

2 onions, chopped

2 tablespoons water

4 cups cooked black beans (2 cups dried, or 2 [14-ounce] cans)

1 (28-ounce) can crushed tomatoes

4 teaspoons chili powder

1½ teaspoons salt, plus additional as needed

1   In a large pot set over medium heat, sauté the onions in the water for about 5 minutes, or until soft.

2   Add the black beans, tomatoes, chili powder, and salt. Bring to a boil. Reduce the heat to low. Simmer for 1 hour, stirring occasionally.

3   Taste, and adjust the seasoning if necessary.

SUBSTITUTION TIP: *Want to skip the tomatoes? Use puréed squash or puréed beets instead. If you omit the chili powder, this won't be chili any more—it will be black bean stew. Toss in some cumin and oregano instead. It will still be delicious!*

PER SERVING Calories: 294; Total Fat: 1g; Total Carbohydrates: 55g; Sugar: 10g; Fiber: 15g; Protein: 18g; Sodium: 858mg

SIMPLE BLACK BEAN SHEPHERD'S PIE

SERVES 4 TO 6   PREP TIME: 10 MINUTES   COOK TIME: 50 MINUTES TO 1 HOUR

CORN FREE
DAIRY FREE
EGG FREE
GLUTEN FREE
NIGHTSHADE FREE
NUT FREE
SOY FREE
VEGAN

This is a hearty recipe that can easily be prepared ahead of time. Once you assemble the shepherd's pie, cover and refrigerator it for up to four days. Then all you need to do is bake it when ready to serve. Alternately, freeze this dish for up to three months.

3 sweet potatoes, cubed

2 tablespoons coconut oil

1 teaspoon salt, divided

1 onion, chopped

2 tablespoons water, plus additional for cooking

3 carrots, grated

2 cups cooked black beans, or 1 (14-ounce) can

1   Preheat the oven to 350°F.

2   Fill a large pot with 2 inches of water and insert a steamer basket. Bring to a boil over high heat.

3   Add the sweet potatoes. Cover and steam for 10 to 12 minutes, or until tender. Drain off any remaining liquid.

4   Add the coconut oil and ½ teaspoon of salt. Mash the sweet potatoes and set aside.

5   In a large skillet set over medium heat, sauté the onion in 2 tablespoons of water for about 5 minutes, or until softened.

6   Add the carrots. Cook for 5 minutes. Remove from the heat.

7   Stir in the black beans and remaining ½ teaspoon of salt. Transfer the mixture to a 9-by-9-inch baking dish.

8   Top with the mashed sweet potatoes.

9   Place the dish in the preheated oven and bake for 30 minutes.

10   Cool for a few minutes before serving.

SUBSTITUTION TIP: *A variety of vegetables can replace sweet potatoes as the topping: mashed winter squash (any variety), carrots, parsnips, celery root, and cauliflower all work beautifully.*

PER SERVING Calories: 431; Total Fat: 8g; Total Carbohydrates: 79g; Sugar: 5g; Fiber: 15g; Protein: 14g; Sodium: 630mg

VEGETABLE SPRING ROLL WRAPS

SERVES 4 TO 6   PREP TIME: 20 MINUTES   COOK TIME: 0 MINUTES

CORN FREE
DAIRY FREE
EGG FREE
GLUTEN FREE
NIGHTSHADE FREE
NUT FREE
SOY FREE
VEGAN

This recipe is great for when you crave something light and fresh, or it's just too hot to cook. Rice paper wrappers can be found in most international sections of grocery stores. These wrappers need to be soaked in warm water for a minute or two to become pliable. The first time you use them, it might take a roll or two before you perfect your wrapping technique. These wraps pair well with the Lemon-Dill Sour Cream (page 183) or Garlic-Tahini Sauce (page 177), but they are also lovely on their own.

10 rice paper wrappers

2 cups lightly packed baby spinach, divided

1 cup grated carrot, divided

1 cucumber, halved, seeded, and cut into thin, 4-inch-long strips, divided

1 avocado, halved, pitted, and cut into thin strips, divided

1   Place a cutting board on a flat surface with the vegetables in front of you.

2   Fill a large, shallow bowl with warm water—hot enough to cook the wrappers, but warm enough so you can touch it comfortably.

3   Soak 1 wrapper in the water and then place it on the cutting board.

4   Fill the middle of the wrapper with ¼ cup of spinach, 2 tablespoons of grated carrot, a few cucumber slices, and 1 or 2 slices of avocado.

5   Fold the sides over the middle, and then roll the wrapper tightly from the bottom (the side closest to you), burrito-style.

6   Repeat with the remaining wrappers and vegetables.

7   Serve immediately.

MAKE AHEAD TIP: *If you aren't serving these right away, the rice paper wrappers will dry out (even if the time between preparing and serving is only an hour). To prevent this, lightly dampen a paper towel or cloth napkin and cover the rolls to keep them moist.*

PER SERVING Calories: 246; Total Fat: 10g; Total Carbohydrates: 36g; Sugar: 4g; Fiber: 6g; Protein: 4g; Sodium: 145mg

TAHINI-KALE NOODLES

SERVES 4   PREP TIME: 5 MINUTES   COOK TIME: 8 TO 10 MINUTES

CORN FREE
DAIRY FREE
EGG FREE
GLUTEN FREE
NIGHTSHADE FREE
NUT FREE
SOY FREE
VEGAN

What constitutes a serving of pasta or noodles? Grab a fistful of noodles between the size of a dime's diameter (1 ounce dry) and a quarter's (2 ounces dry). This recipe is a powerhouse of anti-inflammatory nutrients like amino acids, vitamins C and A, and also includes a payload of calcium.

8 ounces brown rice spaghetti, or buckwheat noodles

4 cups lightly packed kale

½ cup tahini

¾ cup hot water, plus additional as needed

¼ teaspoon salt, plus additional as needed

½ cup chopped fresh parsley

1   Cook the noodles according to the package instructions. During the last 30 seconds of cook time, toss in the kale. In a colander, drain the noodles and kale. Transfer to a large bowl.

2   In a medium bowl, stir together the tahini, hot water, and salt. If you'd like a thinner sauce, add more water.

3   Add the parsley and sauce to the noodles. Toss to coat. Taste, and adjust the seasoning if necessary.

4   Serve hot or cold.

SUBSTITUTION TIP: *Ready for a change from tahini? Use sunflower seed butter, pumpkin seed butter, almond butter, walnut butter, or cashew butter instead.*

PER SERVING Calories: 404; Total Fat: 18g; Total Carbohydrates: 54g; Sugar: 2g; Fiber: 10g; Protein: 15g; Sodium: 223mg

BABY BOK CHOY STIR-FRY

SERVES 6   PREP TIME: 12 MINUTES   COOK TIME: 10 TO 13 MINUTES

CORN FREE
DAIRY FREE
EGG FREE
GLUTEN FREE
NIGHTSHADE FREE
NUT FREE
SOY FREE
PALEO
VEGAN

A member of the cruciferous family, bok choy is a great source of anti-inflammatory nutrients, including vitamins C, A, and K, and omega-3 fatty acids. They have a milder flavor than other crucifers and absorb the additional spices in this stir-fry.

2 tablespoons coconut oil

1 large onion, finely diced

1-inch piece fresh ginger, grated

2 teaspoons ground cumin

1 teaspoon ground turmeric

½ teaspoon salt

12 baby bok choy heads, ends trimmed and sliced lengthwise

Water, as needed for cooking

3 cups cooked brown rice

1   In a large pan set over medium heat, heat the coconut oil.

2   Add the onion and cook for 5 minutes.

3   Add the ginger, cumin, turmeric, and salt. Stir to coat the onion with the spices.

4   Add the bok choy. Stir-fry for 5 to 8 minutes, or until the bok choy is crisp-tender. If the pan gets dry, add 1 tablespoon of water at a time until done.

5   Serve with the brown rice.

INGREDIENT TIP: *If you have extra bok choy in the refrigerator, toss it into your next batch of vegetable broth. It won't overpower the flavor, yet offers a potent punch of nutrients.*

NOTE *that the Week One Plan calls for leftovers; double the quantities so you have enough for later in the week.*

PER SERVING Calories: 444; Total Fat: 9g; Total Carbohydrates: 76g; Sugar: 21g; Fiber: 19g; Protein: 30g; Sodium: 1290mg

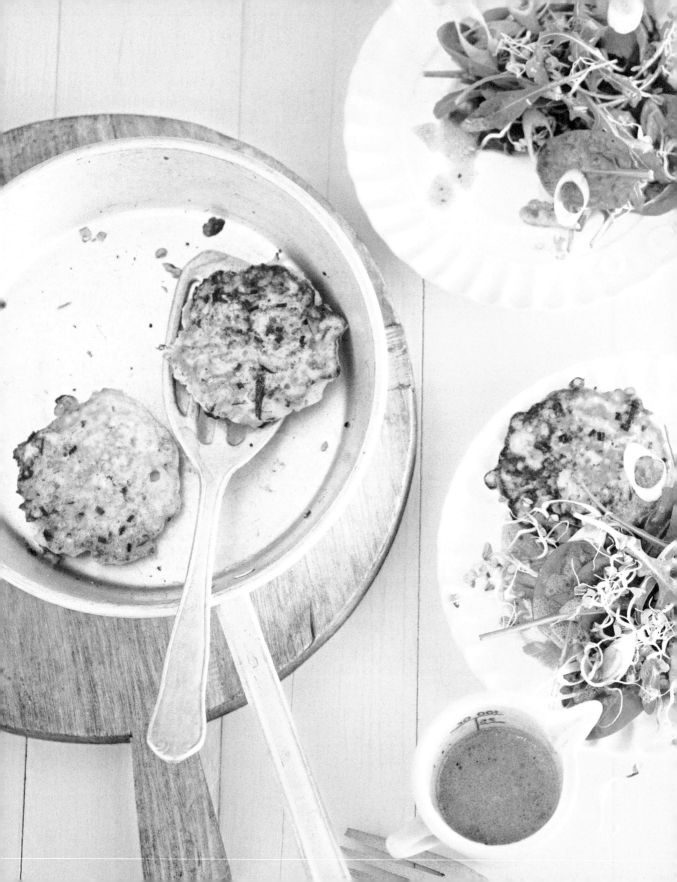

GRAIN-FREE FRITTERS

MAKES 12   PREP TIME: 5 MINUTES   COOK TIME: 20 MINUTES

CORN FREE
DAIRY FREE
EGG FREE
GLUTEN FREE
NIGHTSHADE FREE
NUT FREE
SOY FREE
VEGAN

Fritters or patties can be a challenge when gluten and eggs aren't in the picture. These grain-free fritters are easy to make, hold together well, and have a surprisingly eggy flavor. There are two keys to their success: use medium-low heat to cook the fritters gently and evenly, and don't flip the fritters too soon. After dolloping batter into the pan, resist the instinct to slide the spatula under the fritters just to "check if they're sticking." This is how you end up with a goopy mess and a frown on your face. Give the fritters due time to cook, and you will be rewarded with crunchy, crispy treats. Pair with a Simple Spinach Salad (page 98) for a light lunch or dinner.

2 cups chickpea flour

1½ cups water

2 tablespoons chia seeds, ground

½ teaspoon salt

3 cups lightly packed spinach leaves, finely chopped

1 tablespoon coconut oil, or extra-virgin olive oil

1   In a medium bowl, whisk together the chickpea flour, water, chia seeds, and salt. Mix well to ensure there are no lumps.

2   Fold in the spinach.

3   In a nonstick skillet set over medium-low heat, melt the coconut oil. »

4   Working in batches, use a ¼-cup measure to drop the batter into the pan. Flatten the fritters to about ½ inch thick. Don't crowd the pan.

5   Cook for 5 to 6 minutes. Flip the fritters and cook for 5 minutes more.

6   Transfer to a serving plate.

SUBSTITUTION TIP: *Any dark leafy green can be substituted here cup for cup for the spinach. Also try broccoli, zucchini, carrots, and sweet potatoes or add extra spices like ground ginger, cumin, turmeric, coriander, dried basil, oregano, or rosemary.*

PER SERVING (2 fritters) Calories: 318; Total Fat: 10g; Total Carbohydrates: 45g; Sugar: 7g; Fiber: 15g; Protein: 15g; Sodium: 222mg

HOMEMADE AVOCADO SUSHI

SERVES 4   PREP TIME: 20 MINUTES   COOK TIME: 15 MINUTES

CORN FREE
DAIRY FREE
EGG FREE
GLUTEN FREE
NIGHTSHADE FREE
NUT FREE
SOY FREE
VEGAN

Sushi is easy to make at home and you don't need any special equipment like bamboo mats or chopsticks. The only unusual ingredient you'll need is nori sheets, which are readily available nowadays in the international section of most supermarkets. Most sushi is prepared with white rice; I usually use quinoa.

1½ cups dry quinoa

3 cups water, plus additional for rolling

½ teaspoon salt

6 nori sheets

3 avocados, halved, pitted, and sliced thin, divided

1 small cucumber, halved, seeded, and cut into matchsticks, divided

Coconut aminos, for dipping (optional)

1   Rinse the quinoa in a fine-mesh sieve.

2   In a medium pot set over high heat, combine the rinsed quinoa, water, and salt. Bring to a boil. Reduce the heat to low. Cover and simmer for 15 minutes. Fluff the quinoa with a fork.

3   On a cutting board, lay out 1 nori sheet. Spread ½ cup of quinoa over the sheet, leaving 2 to 3 inches uncovered at the top.

4   Place 5 or 6 avocado slices across the bottom of the nori sheet (the side closest to you) in a row. Add 5 or 6 cucumber matchsticks on top.

5   Starting at the bottom, tightly roll up the nori sheet. sheet. Dab the uncovered top with water to seal the roll.

6   Slice the sushi roll into 6 pieces.

7   Repeat with the remaining 5 nori sheets, quinoa, and vegetables.

8   Serve with the coconut aminos (if using).

INGREDIENT TIP: *Coconut aminos, derived from coconuts, mimics the taste of soy sauce. It can be difficult to locate and is often expensive. Another option for dipping is fish sauce or tahini.*

PER SERVING Calories: 557; Total Fat: 33g; Total Carbohydrates: 57g; Sugar: 2g; Fiber: 15g; Protein: 13g; Sodium: 309mg

HOME-STYLE RED LENTIL STEW

SERVES 6   PREP TIME: 10 MINUTES   COOK TIME: 35 MINUTES

Like all lentils, the red variety is packed with protein, fiber, B vitamins, and energy-boosting iron. What differentiates red lentils from its siblings, other than its bright red-orange color, is the super-quick cooking time. Red lentils are so little they disintegrate as they cook, yielding a thick, stick-to-your-ribs texture that doesn't need blending. Hooray for one less step!

2 onions, peeled and finely diced

4 celery stalks, finely diced

6½ cups plus 2 tablespoons water, divided

3 cups red lentils

2 zucchini, finely diced

1 teaspoon dried oregano

1 teaspoon salt, plus additional as needed

1   In a large pot set over medium heat, sauté the onions and celery in 2 tablespoons of water for about 5 minutes, or until soft.

2   Add the lentils, zucchini, the remaining 6½ cups of water, the oregano, and salt. Bring to a boil. Reduce the heat to low. Cover and simmer for 30 minutes, stirring occasionally.

3   Taste, and adjust the seasoning if necessary.

SUBSTITUTION TIP: *If you enjoy this recipe, try it with different types of lentils. However, brown or green lentils will need additional cooking time, at least 15 minutes.*

NOTE *that the Week Two Plan calls for leftovers; double the quantities so you have enough for later in the week.*

PER SERVING Calories: 367; Total Fat: 1g; Total Carbohydrates: 64g; Sugar: 5g; Fiber: 31g; Protein: 26g; Sodium: 410mg

BROCCOLI and BEAN CASSEROLE

SERVES 4   PREP TIME: 10 MINUTES   COOK TIME: 35 TO 40 MINUTES

CORN FREE
DAIRY FREE
EGG FREE
GLUTEN FREE
NIGHTSHADE FREE
SOY FREE
VEGAN

Don't toss out those broccoli stalks. They contain the same nutrients as the florets and they taste the same, too. I peel and chop the stalks and add them to a variety of dishes, especially soups, stews, and casseroles. You can also freeze them to use later when making soup stock.

¾ cup vegetable broth, or water

2 broccoli heads, crowns and stalks finely chopped

1 teaspoon salt

2 cups cooked pinto or navy beans, or 1 (14-ounce) can

1 to 2 tablespoons brown rice flour, or arrowroot flour

1 cup walnuts, chopped

1   Preheat the oven to 350°F.

2   In a large ovenproof pot set over medium heat, warm the broth.

3   Add the broccoli and salt. Cook for 6 to 8 minutes, or until the broccoli is bright green.

4   Stir in the pinto beans and brown rice flour. Cook for 5 minutes more, or until the liquid thickens slightly.

5   Sprinkle the walnuts over the top.

6   Place the pot in the preheated oven and bake for 20 to 25 minutes. The walnuts should be toasted.

SUBSTITUTION TIP: *If nut allergies are an issue, use sunflower seeds or pumpkin seeds to replace the walnuts. If you're not a fan of walnuts, use any nut you love.*

PER SERVING Calories: 410; Total Fat: 20g; Total Carbohydrates: 43g; Sugar: 4g; Fiber: 13g; Protein: 22g; Sodium: 635mg

BROWN RICE PASTA with CREAMY CARROT "MARINARA"

SERVES 6 PREP TIME: 15 MINUTES COOK TIME: 20 MINUTES

CORN FREE
DAIRY FREE
EGG FREE
GLUTEN FREE
NIGHTSHADE FREE
SOY FREE
VEGAN

A nightshade-free life doesn't mean you have to give up marinara. This version uses carrots as the base, and is so thick, creamy, and luxurious you'll want to top everything with it. If you have additional herbs on hand, like fresh or dried parsley, oregano, or thyme, toss them in as well.

1¼ cups cashews, soaked in water for at least 4 hours

5 large carrots, peeled and roughly chopped

1½ to 2 cups water

1 tablespoon finely chopped fresh basil

1 teaspoon salt

1 (12-ounce) package brown rice spaghetti

1 bunch kale, thoroughly washed, stemmed, and chopped into 1-inch pieces

1   Drain and rinse the cashews.

2   In a medium pot set over high heat, combine the carrots with 1½ cups of water. Bring to a boil. Reduce the heat to low and simmer for 5 to 8 minutes, or until tender. Drain the carrots and reserve the cooking water.

3   In a blender, combine the cashews, basil, and salt. Add the cooked carrots and reserved cooking water. Blend until smooth, taking care with the hot liquid. If the sauce is too thick, thin with more water.

4 Bring a large pot of water to a boil over high heat. Add the pasta and cook according to the package directions.

5 During the last minute of cook time, toss in the kale and let it wilt. Drain the pasta and return it to the pot. Toss with the carrot marinara. You may not need to use all of the sauce. Leftover sauce will keep refrigerated for 3 to 4 days, and freezes well.

SUBSTITUTION TIP: *If nut allergies are a problem, substitute soaked sunflower seeds or sesame seeds.*

NOTE *that the Week One Plan calls for leftovers; double the quantities so you have enough for later in the week.*

PER SERVING Calories: 408; Total Fat: 14g; Total Carbohydrates: 65g; Sugar: 4g; Fiber: 4g; Protein: 10g; Sodium: 460mg

BUCKWHEAT-VEGETABLE POLENTA

SERVES 6   PREP TIME: 15 MINUTES   COOK TIME: 20 MINUTES

Miss creamy polenta? You won't when buckwheat is around. This special, magnesium-rich fruit seed has a consistency similar to polenta when ground into meal. This vegetable polenta isn't "traditional," but it is delicious.

3 cups buckwheat

¼ cup extra-virgin olive oil

6 garlic cloves, minced

7 to 8 cups warm vegetable broth (homemade or purchased), divided

2 cups shredded zucchini

6 cups spinach, finely chopped

1 teaspoon salt, plus additional as needed

1   In a spice grinder, high-speed blender, or food processor, grind the buckwheat until fine.

2   In a large pot set over medium-low heat, heat the olive oil. Add the garlic and sauté for 3 minutes.

3   Add the ground buckwheat and stir to coat with the garlic and oil.

4   Stir in 1 cup of vegetable broth. When all the liquid is absorbed, add another 1 cup of broth, along with the zucchini and spinach. Repeat with the remaining 4 cups of broth, 1 cup at a time, until the buckwheat is tender and the consistency of a thick polenta. You may not need to use all the broth.

5   Add the salt. Stir, taste, and adjust the seasoning if necessary.

SUBSTITUTION TIP: *If you and your dinner mates are not vegetarian, use Basic Chicken Broth (page 93) instead. You can even make this recipe with plain water, but you might need to add some additional salt and herbs for flavor.*

NOTE *that the Week One Plan calls for leftovers; double the quantities so you have enough for later in the week.*

PER SERVING Calories: 426; Total Fat: 13g; Total Carbohydrates: 65g; Sugar: 2g; Fiber: 10g; Protein: 18g; Sodium: 1307mg

QUINOA FLATBREAD PIZZA

SERVES 4 TO 6   PREP TIME: 10 MINUTES   COOK TIME: 40 MINUTES,
INCLUDES 25 MINUTES QUINOA FLATBREAD COOKING TIME

CORN FREE
DAIRY FREE
EGG FREE
GLUTEN FREE
NIGHTSHADE FREE
NUT FREE
SOY FREE
VEGAN

The quinoa flatbread used in this recipe is going to become your favorite pizza crust of all time. It's thin yet hearty, and stands up well to toppings. What I use here are some simple topping suggestions. If you've got more vegetables and herbs in the refrigerator that need to be used, pile them on. This crust can take it.

1 Quinoa Flatbread (page 76)

1 cup pearl onions, halved

2 tablespoons extra-virgin olive oil

2 cups arugula

1 (14-ounce) can artichoke hearts in water

2 tablespoons pine nuts (optional)

1   Prepare the flatbread according to the recipe's instructions. When the flatbread is done, remove it from the oven and increase the heat to 375°F.

2   In a small baking dish, toss together the pearl onions and olive oil.

3   Place the dish in the preheated oven and roast for 10 minutes.

4   Scatter the onions over the crust.

5   Top with the arugula, artichoke hearts, and pine nuts (if using).

6   Place the pizza back in the oven and bake for 12 minutes.

7   Cool the pizza slightly before slicing and serving.

MAKE AHEAD TIP: *The crust can be made ahead of time. Allow it to cool completely, then wrap tightly in parchment paper. Refrigerate if using in the next few days, or place it in a resealable plastic freezer bag and freeze for another time.*

SUBSTITUTION TIP: *If you're fine with nightshades and want to eat them after the elimination diet, use homemade or purchased tomato sauce. This recipe is also amazing with pesto, Creamy Carrot Marinara (page 116), or hummus as the sauce.*

PER SERVING Calories: 181; Total Fat: 13g; Total Carbohydrates: 13g; Sugar: 2g; Fiber: 2g; Protein: 4g; Sodium: 407mg

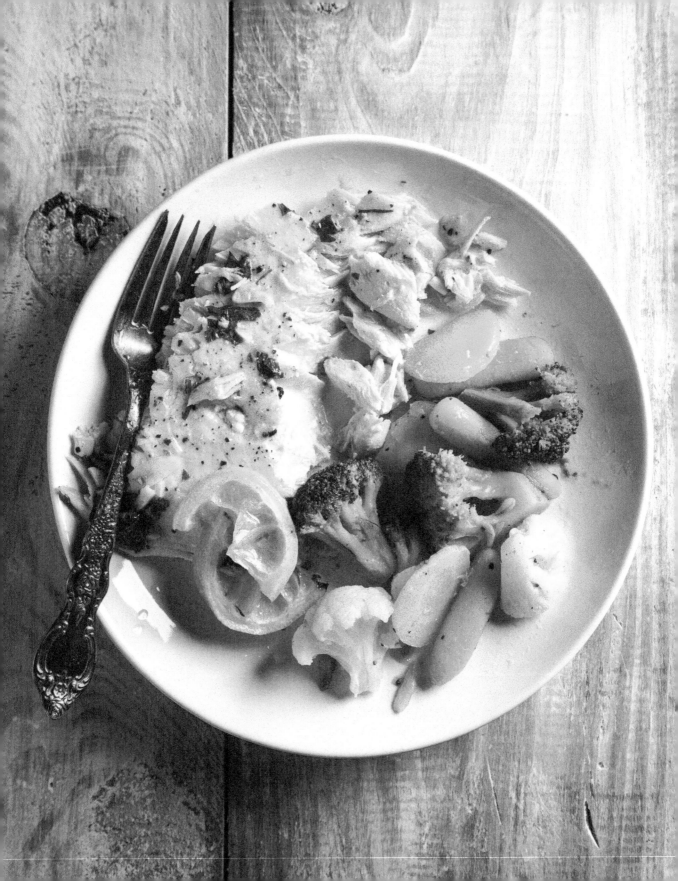

SEAFOOD DISHES

7

LEMONY SALMON with MIXED VEGETABLES

SERVES 4   PREP TIME: 10 MINUTES   COOK TIME: 25 TO 30 MINUTES

CORN FREE
DAIRY FREE
EGG FREE
GLUTEN FREE
NIGHTSHADE FREE
NUT FREE
SOY FREE
PALEO

There is something about the pairing of wild salmon and lemon that is so fresh and appealing. Aside from its delicious taste, the salmon's anti-inflammatory omega-3 fats will help you better absorb the nutrients in the vegetables—particularly the vitamin C. How's that for a power couple?

4 (5-ounce) wild salmon fillets

1 teaspoon salt, divided

1 lemon, washed and sliced thin

1 broccoli head, roughly chopped

1 cauliflower head, roughly chopped

1 small bunch (4 to 6) carrots, cut into coins

1   Preheat the oven to 400°F.

2   Line a baking sheet with parchment paper.

3   Place the salmon on the prepared sheet.

4   Sprinkle the salmon with ½ teaspoon of salt. Drape each fillet with a few lemon slices.

5   Place the sheet in the preheated oven and bake for 15 to 20 minutes, or until the salmon is opaque and flakes easily with a fork.

6   While the salmon cooks, fill a pot with 3 inches of water and insert a steamer basket. Bring to a boil over high heat.

7   Add the broccoli, cauliflower, and carrots to the pot. Cover and cook for 8 to 10 minutes.

8   Sprinkle with the remaining ½ teaspoon of salt.

9   Top each salmon fillet with a heaping pile of vegetables, and serve.

SUBSTITUTION TIP: *Broccoli, cauliflower, and carrots create a simple, inexpensive side dish, but you can use any of your favorite vegetables to complement the salmon. Sweet potatoes or beets work well, or pair the salmon with any variety of fresh or steamed greens.*

PER SERVING Calories: 330; Total Fat: 13g; Total Carbohydrates: 20g; Sugar: 8g; Fiber: 7g; Protein: 35g; Sodium: 761mg

SARDINE DONBURI

SERVES 4 TO 6   PREP TIME: 10 MINUTES   COOK TIME: 45 TO 50 MINUTES

CORN FREE
DAIRY FREE
EGG FREE
GLUTEN FREE
NIGHTSHADE FREE
NUT FREE
SOY FREE

Sardines get a bad rap and I can't figure out why. They're not gross or stinky—in fact, I find them far less odorous than the ever-popular tuna. Sardines are an amazing source of anti-inflammatory omega-3 fats, protein, and bone-building vitamin D and calcium.

2 cups brown rice, rinsed well

4 cups water

½ teaspoon salt

3 (4-ounce) cans sardines packed in water, drained

3 scallions, sliced thin

1-inch piece fresh ginger, grated

4 tablespoons sesame oil, or extra-virgin olive oil, divided

1   In a large pot, combine the rice, water, and salt. Bring to a boil over high heat. Reduce the heat to low. Cover and cook for 45 to 50 minutes, or until tender.

2   In a medium bowl, roughly mash the sardines.

3   When the rice is done, add the sardines, scallions, and ginger to the pot. Mix thoroughly.

4   Divide the rice among four bowls. Drizzle each bowl with 1 teaspoon to 1 tablespoon of sesame oil.

SUBSTITUTION TIP: *Don't have the time to wait for brown rice to cook? Use quinoa or buckwheat instead, as these will cook in 15 to 20 minutes.*

PER SERVING Calories: 604; Total Fat: 24g; Total Carbohydrates: 74g; Sugar: 0g; Fiber: 4g; Protein: 25g; Sodium: 499mg

TASTY FISH TACOS with PINEAPPLE SALSA

SERVES 6   PREP TIME: 15 MINUTES   COOK TIME: 12 MINUTES

CORN FREE
DAIRY FREE
EGG FREE
GLUTEN FREE
NIGHTSHADE FREE
NUT FREE
SOY FREE
PALEO

These simple tacos are a fresh, tasty option any time of year, but there's something about them that just screams "summer." If you have access to a barbecue or countertop grill, you can grill the fish—and the pineapple, too—which will take the salsa to the next flavor level. Choose large pineapple pieces or rings so they don't fall through the grill.

FOR THE SALSA

1½ cups fresh, or canned, pineapple chunks, cut into small dice

1 small red onion, minced

Juice of 1 lime

Zest of 1 lime

FOR THE TACOS

1 head romaine lettuce

3 tablespoons coconut oil

14 ounces white fish, skinless and firm, such as cod or halibut

Juice of 1 lime

Zest of 1 lime

½ teaspoon salt

TO MAKE THE SALSA

In a medium bowl, stir together the pineapple and onion. Add the lime juice and lime zest. Stir well and set aside.

TO MAKE THE TACOS

1   Separate the lettuce leaves, choosing the 6 to 12 largest and most suitable to hold the filling. Wash the leaves and pat them dry.

2   In a large pan set over medium-low heat, heat the coconut oil.

3   Brush the fish with the lime juice and lime zest. Sprinkle with the salt.

4   Place the fish in the pan. Cook for 8 minutes.

5   Flip the fish over and break it up into small pieces. Cook for 3 to 4 minutes more. The flesh should be opaque and flake easily with a fork.

6   Fill the lettuce leaves with the cooked fish (double the leaves for extra strength), and spoon the salsa over the top.

MAKE AHEAD TIP: *Prepare the salsa a day ahead for convenience and extra flavor.*

PER SERVING Calories: 198; Total Fat: 9g; Total Carbohydrates: 12g; Sugar: 8g; Fiber: 2g; Protein: 19g; Sodium: 245mg

WHITEFISH CHOWDER

SERVES 6 TO 8   PREP TIME: 10 MINUTES   COOK TIME: 35 MINUTES

Coconut milk lends this minimalist chowder its delicious creaminess. Use the full-fat variety, as it will add a satisfying thickness to your bowl. If you have any extra anti-inflammatory vegetables kicking around in the refrigerator, throw them in, too.

4 carrots, peeled and cut into ½-inch pieces

3 sweet potatoes, peeled and cut into ½-inch pieces

3 cups full-fat coconut milk

2 cups water

1 teaspoon dried thyme

½ teaspoon salt

10½ ounces white fish, skinless and firm, such as cod or halibut, cut into chunks

1   In a large pot, combine the carrots, sweet potatoes, coconut milk, water, thyme, and salt. Bring to a boil over high heat. Reduce the heat to low. Cover and simmer for 20 minutes.

2   In a blender, purée half of the soup. Return the purée to the pot. Add the fish chunks.

3   Cook for 12 to 15 minutes more, or until the fish is tender and hot.

SUBSTITUTION TIP: *If you don't like the taste of coconut milk, substitute almond milk. To achieve the same creamy texture, blend three-fourths of the soup before returning it to the pot.*

NOTE *that the Week One Plan calls for leftovers; double the quantities so you have enough for later in the week.*

PER SERVING Calories: 451; Total Fat: 29g; Total Carbohydrates: 39g; Sugar: 7g; Fiber: 8g; Protein: 14g; Sodium: 251mg

CAULIFLOWER and COD STEW

SERVES 4   PREP TIME: 15 MINUTES   COOK TIME: 30 MINUTES

CORN FREE
DAIRY FREE
EGG FREE
GLUTEN FREE
NIGHTSHADE FREE
SOY FREE
PALEO

The combination of cooked cauliflower and cashews is rich, delicious, and comforting. This recipe is a riff on Slow-Cooker Chicken Alfredo (page 153), and the cauliflower base pairs wonderfully with the cod (also known as the fish in fish 'n' chips!). If you're not a fan of cod, substitute another white fish that strikes your fancy.

3 cups water

1 large cauliflower head, broken into large florets (about 4 cups)

1 cup cashews, soaked in water for at least 4 hours

1 teaspoon salt

1 pound cod, cut into chunks

2 cups kale, thoroughly washed and sliced

1. In a large pot set over high heat, bring the water to a boil. Reduce the heat to medium.

2. Add the cauliflower. Cook for 12 minutes, or until tender.

3. Drain and rinse the cashews and place them in a blender.

4. Add the cooked cauliflower and its cooking water to the blender.

5. Add the salt.

6. Blend until smooth, adding more water if you prefer a thinner consistency.

7. Return the blended cauliflower-cashew mixture to the pot. Place the pot over medium heat.

8. Add the cod. Cook for about 15 minutes, or until cooked through.

9. Add the kale. Let it wilt for about 3 minutes.

SUBSTITUTION TIP: *If nut allergies are a concern, substitute soaked sunflower seeds in place of the cashews.*

PER SERVING Calories: 385; Total Fat: 17g; Total Carbohydrates: 26g; Sugar: 7g; Fiber: 7g; Protein: 36g; Sodium: 753mg

SAUTÉED SARDINES with CAULIFLOWER MASH

SERVES 4   PREP TIME: 10 MINUTES   COOK TIME: 15 MINUTES

CORN FREE
DAIRY FREE
EGG FREE
GLUTEN FREE
NIGHTSHADE FREE
SOY FREE
PALEO

Miss mashed potatoes? Meet mashed cauliflower, your soon-to-be new food obsession. When steamed and mashed, cauliflower has a texture and taste remarkably similar to mashed potatoes. For extra creaminess, add 1 to 2 tablespoons of your favorite nondairy milk, or add chives, rosemary, or roasted garlic.

2 heads cauliflower, broken into large florets

4 tablespoons extra-virgin olive oil, divided

¼ teaspoon salt

4 (4-ounce) cans sardines packed in water, drained

1 cup fresh parsley, finely chopped

1   Fill a large pot with 2 inches of water and insert a steamer basket. Bring the water to a boil over high heat.

2   Add the cauliflower to the basket. Cover and steam for 8 to 10 minutes, or until the florets are tender. Transfer the cauliflower to a food processor.

3   Add 2 tablespoons of olive oil and the salt to the cauliflower. Process until the cauliflower is smooth and creamy. Depending on the size of your processor, you may need to do this in two batches.

4   In a medium bowl, roughly mash the sardines.

5   Add the remaining 2 tablespoons of olive oil to a medium pan set over low heat. When oil is shimmering, add the sardines and parsley. Cook for 3 minutes. You want the sardines to be warm, not scalding hot.

6   Serve the sardines with a generous scoop of cauliflower mash.

COOKING TIP: *If you're feeling lazy and don't want to wash another piece of equipment, skip the food processor. Put the cooked cauliflower in a bowl and use a potato masher instead.*

PER SERVING Calories: 334; Total Fat: 24g; Total Carbohydrates: 8g; Sugar: 3g; Fiber: 4g; Protein: 26g; Sodium: 465mg

BAKED SALMON PATTIES with GREENS

SERVES 4   PREP TIME: 15 MINUTES   COOK TIME: 35 TO 38 MINUTES

CORN FREE
DAIRY FREE
EGG FREE
GLUTEN FREE
NIGHTSHADE FREE
SOY FREE
PALEO

I was never a big fan of fish as a kid, but I made an exception for salmon patties—a staple meal back then. This version is made without eggs, and has the added benefit of anti-inflammatory sweet potatoes and turmeric. My grandmother insisted that my mother make them using canned salmon with bones, as the bones are a good source of calcium. This is advice I follow today. If you find the bones unpalatable, use boneless canned salmon.

2 cups cooked, mashed sweet potatoes (about 2 large sweet potatoes)

2 (6-ounce) cans wild salmon, drained

¼ cup almond flour

¼ teaspoon ground turmeric

2 tablespoons coconut oil

2 kale bunches, thoroughly washed, stemmed, and cut into ribbons

¼ teaspoon salt

1   Preheat the oven to 350°F.

2   Line a baking sheet with parchment paper.

3   In a large bowl, stir together the mashed sweet potatoes and salmon.

4   Blend in the almond flour and turmeric.

5   Using a ⅓-cup measure, scoop the salmon mixture onto the baking sheet. Flatten slightly with the bottom of the measuring cup. Repeat with the remaining mixture.

6   Place the sheet in the preheated oven and bake for 30 minutes, flipping the patties halfway through.

7   In a large pan set over medium heat, heat the coconut oil.

8   Add the kale. Sauté for 5 to 8 minutes, or until the kale is bright and wilted. Sprinkle with the salt and serve with the salmon patties.

SUBSTITUTION TIP: *To make this recipe nut-free, in a spice grinder or blender, grind 3 tablespoons of sunflower seeds to a fine meal.*

PER SERVING Calories: 320; Total Fat: 13g; Total Carbohydrates: 32g; Sugar: 0g; Fiber: 5g; Protein: 21g; Sodium: 88mg

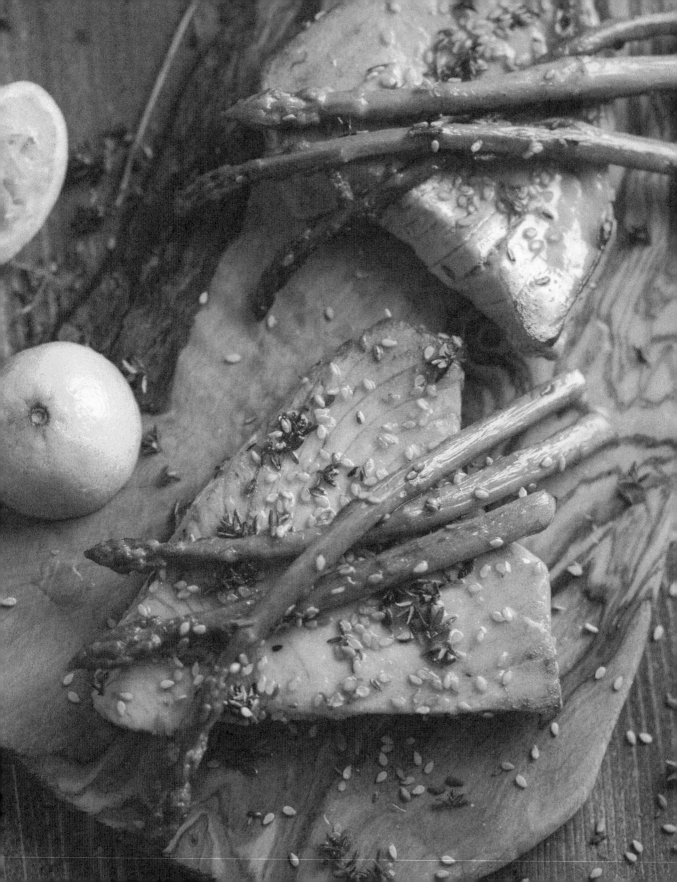

SESAME-TUNA with ASPARAGUS

SERVES 4   PREP TIME: 10 MINUTES   COOK TIME: 15 MINUTES

CORN FREE
DAIRY FREE
EGG FREE
GLUTEN FREE
NIGHTSHADE FREE
NUT FREE
SOY FREE
PALEO

Most people are accustomed to eating tuna from cans rather than fresh fillets. A tuna steak seems fancy while canned tuna seems a more accessible, run-of-the-mill option. Tuna fillets are quick and simple to cook, creating an elegant and extremely healthy meal. Like other kinds of fish, tuna is rich in omega-3s, but it also contains a wide span of nutrients like stress-busting B vitamins, magnesium, potassium, and selenium. You won't be sorry if you try this!

2 asparagus bunches, washed and trimmed

3 tablespoons toasted sesame oil, divided

½ teaspoon salt

4 (4-ounce) tuna steaks

2 tablespoons sesame seeds

1   Preheat the oven to 375°F.

2   Line a baking sheet with parchment paper.

3   In a large bowl, combine the asparagus, 1½ tablespoons of sesame oil, and the salt. Spread the asparagus onto the prepared sheet.

4   Place the sheet in the preheated oven and bake for 15 minutes.

5   While the asparagus cooks, brush the tuna with the remaining 1½ tablespoons of sesame oil.

6   Place a sauté pan over medium heat. When the pan is hot, add the tuna. Depending on the size of your pan, you may need to cook the tuna steaks one or two at a time.

7   Sear the tuna for 3 to 4 minutes on each side, or longer if you like your tuna more well done.

8   Plate the tuna and the asparagus on four plates. Sprinkle 1½ teaspoons of sesame seeds over each serving.

PREPARATION TIP: *Snap off the woody bottoms of asparagus spears; they have a natural breaking point that guides which part should be discarded. Simply bend the spears toward the bottom until they give way and split.*

PER SERVING Calories: 349; Total Fat: 20g; Total Carbohydrates: 6g; Sugar: 2g; Fiber: 3g; Protein: 37g; Sodium: 350mg

CURRY-GLAZED SALMON with QUINOA

SERVES 6   PREP TIME: 10 MINUTES   COOK TIME: 30 TO 35 MINUTES

CORN FREE
DAIRY FREE
EGG FREE
GLUTEN FREE
NIGHTSHADE FREE
NUT FREE
SOY FREE

Curry powder is a blend of anti-inflammatory spices including cumin, coriander, turmeric, ginger, cardamom, and more. It also contains chiles, so spice levels of different curry powders may vary. For a chile-free version, make your own curry powder and omit the chiles. There are many recipes online and it makes a fun weekend cooking project.

¼ cup liquid honey

1 teaspoon curry powder, plus additional as needed

6 (4-ounce) wild salmon fillets

2 cups quinoa, rinsed well

4 cups water

½ teaspoon salt

1   Preheat the oven to 350°F.

2   Line a baking sheet with parchment paper.

3   In a small bowl, mix together the honey and curry powder. Taste, and add more curry powder if needed.

4   Pat the fillets dry with a clean kitchen towel and place them on the prepared sheet.

5   Brush the fillets with the curry and honey mixture.

6   In a medium pot, combine the quinoa, water, and salt. Bring to a boil over high heat. Reduce the heat to low. Cover and cook for 15 minutes.

7   Put the salmon into the preheated oven and bake for 15 to 20 minutes, or until the flesh is opaque and flakes easily with a fork.

8   Fluff the quinoa and serve alongside the salmon.

INGREDIENT TIP: *To ensure you are eating sustainable seafood that will maintain the future health of our oceans, check out the websites for Ocean Wise, SeaChoice, or Seafood Watch. These sites contain valuable recommendations of sustainable seafood varieties, along with regions from which to choose fish.*

PER SERVING Calories: 445; Total Fat: 13g; Total Carbohydrates: 48g; Sugar: 12g; Fiber: 4g; Protein: 32g; Sodium: 251mg

MACKEREL RISOTTO

SERVES 4 TO 6   PREP TIME: 10 MINUTES   COOK TIME: 35 MINUTES

Risotto is the type of dish that requires your presence in front of the stove, but all you need to do is stir, so the task isn't too onerous. Pass the time by listening to a podcast or your favorite music, or have a good old-fashioned conversation.

8 cups Basic Chicken Broth (page 93), or vegetable broth

2 tablespoons coconut oil

1 onion, finely diced

4 garlic cloves, minced

2 cups buckwheat

4 (4-ounce) cans Wild Atlantic, King, or Spanish mackerel, drained

½ teaspoon salt (optional)

1   In a large pot set over medium heat, warm the broth.

2   In a second large pot set over medium heat, heat the coconut oil.

3   Add the onion and garlic. Sauté for about 5 minutes, or until soft.

4   Add the buckwheat to the pot and stir for 2 minutes to toast.

5   Add the warm broth, 1 cup at a time, stirring occasionally. When all the liquid is absorbed, add another 1 cup of broth. Repeat until the buckwheat is cooked and tender, about 25 minutes.

6   In a medium bowl, gently mash the mackerel to break it up. Fold the mackerel into the buckwheat.

7   Taste and add the salt (if using).

INGREDIENT TIP: *If you have extra greens in the refrigerator, toss them into this recipe, too. You can never go wrong with an extra burst of vitamins and minerals.*

PER SERVING Calories: 594; Total Fat: 31g; Total Carbohydrates: 36g; Sugar: 3g; Fiber: 5g; Protein: 43g; Sodium: 1231mg

SALMON and MUSHROOM HASH with HERBED PESTO

SERVES 6   PREP TIME: 15 MINUTES   COOK TIME: 20 MINUTES

CORN FREE
DAIRY FREE
EGG FREE
GLUTEN FREE
NIGHTSHADE FREE
NUT FREE
SOY FREE
PALEO

Mushrooms are incredible immune boosters, particularly shiitake and cremini. So add whatever variety you prefer to this dish. Traditional cooking advice says mushrooms should not be washed, but rather wiped clean with a damp kitchen towel or paper towel. I think that takes too long! And, a few years ago, I read an interview with a classically trained French chef who declared that wiping mushrooms was a waste of time and washing them didn't compromise their texture. If it's good enough for a French chef, it's good enough for me.

FOR THE PESTO

1 bunch fresh basil

¼ cup extra-virgin olive oil

Juice of 1 lemon

Zest of 1 lemon

⅓ cup water

¼ teaspoon salt, plus additional as needed

FOR THE HASH

2 tablespoons extra-virgin olive oil, or coconut oil

6 cups mixed mushrooms (brown, white, shiitake, cremini, portobello, etc.), washed, stemmed, and sliced

1 pound wild salmon, cubed

TO MAKE THE PESTO

In a food processor or blender, combine the basil (stems and all), olive oil, lemon juice, lemon zest, water, and salt. Blend until smooth.

TO MAKE THE HASH

1. In a large skillet or pot set over medium heat, heat the olive oil.

2. Add the mushrooms. Cook for 6 to 8 minutes, or until they wilt and start to exude their juices.

3. Add the salmon to the pan. Cook for 10 to 12 minutes more, or until the salmon is cooked through.

4. Stir in the pesto. Taste, and adjust the seasoning if necessary.

EQUIPMENT TIP: *Buy a separate cutting board to chop, slice, or handle meat and fish products. This reduces the risk of cross-contamination in the kitchen.*

PER SERVING Calories: 265; Total Fat: 15g; Total Carbohydrates: 31g; Sugar: 7g; Fiber: 4g; Protein: 7g; Sodium: 481mg

HERBED TUNA CAKES

SERVES 4   PREP TIME: 15 MINUTES   COOK TIME: 30 MINUTES

Affectionately known as the "blonde carrot," parsnips are closely related to carrots, parsley, and celery. They are slightly sweeter than carrots, high in fiber, and contain a number of anti-inflammatory nutrients. Parsnips offer a sweet contrast to the briny flavor of canned tuna in these patties that you'll truly enjoy.

2 cups cooked and mashed parsnips

2 (6-ounce) cans wild tuna, drained

¼ cup almond flour, or brown rice flour

2 tablespoons ground flaxseed, or ground chia seed

1 bunch fresh parsley, stemmed and finely chopped

1   Preheat the oven to 350°F.

2   Line a baking sheet with parchment paper.

3   In a medium bowl, combine the mashed parsnips and tuna, flaking the tuna with a fork.

4   Stir in the almond flour, flaxseed, and parsley. Mix well.

5   Using a ⅓-cup measure, scoop the patty mixture onto the prepared sheet. Flatten slightly with the bottom of the measuring cup. Repeat with the remaining mixture.

6   Place the sheet in the preheated oven and bake for 30 minutes, flipping the patties halfway through.

SERVING TIP: *These tuna cakes are great fresh out of the oven, but they're also delicious chilled. Crumble them over a salad, tuck them into a lettuce wrap, or eat them over a pile of steamed greens. And don't limit yourself to just lunch and dinner; they make a satisfying breakfast, too (and they're portable, so you can take them on the go).*

PER SERVING Calories: 273; Total Fat: 9g; Total Carbohydrates: 23g; Sugar: 4g; Fiber: 5g; Protein: 25g; Sodium: 61mg

ALMOND-CRUSTED HONEY-DIJON SALMON with GREENS

SERVES 6   PREP TIME: 15 MINUTES   COOK TIME: 20 MINUTES

Almond-crusted honey-Dijon salmon sounds fancy, yet this elegant meal is ridiculously simple to make. It's a great meal when you want to impress, but it also makes an easy weeknight dinner.

¾ cup whole almonds

⅓ cup Dijon mustard, plus additional as needed

3 tablespoons raw honey, plus additional as needed

6 (4-ounce) wild salmon fillets

2 tablespoons coconut oil

3 bunches Swiss chard, washed, stemmed, and roughly chopped

½ teaspoon salt

1   Preheat the oven to 350°F.

2   Line a baking sheet with parchment paper.

3   Using a food processor, high-speed blender, or spice grinder, pulverize the almonds into a fine meal. If you are using a spice grinder, you may want to roughly chop the nuts first.

4   In a small bowl, stir together the mustard and honey. Taste and add more honey or mustard, if desired.

5   Put the salmon fillets on the prepared sheet. Gently pat them dry with a paper towel or clean kitchen towel.

6   Brush each fillet with the honey-Dijon mixture.

7   Sprinkle each fillet evenly with 3 tablespoons of almond meal and gently press it into the fillet with the back of a spoon or your hands. If you have any leftover almond meal, refrigerate it for another use.

8   Place the salmon in the preheated oven and bake for 15 to 20 minutes, or until the flesh is opaque and flakes easily with a fork. »

9   While the salmon is cooking, heat the coconut oil in a large pan set over medium heat.

10   Add the Swiss chard. Sauté for 5 to 6 minutes, or until it is bright green and wilted. Sprinkle with the salt.

11   Remove the salmon from the oven and serve with the greens.

SUBSTITUTION TIP: *Make this nut-free by substituting coconut instead of the almonds. Use ½ to ¾ cup unsweetened shredded coconut as the crust for the salmon.*

COOKING TIP: *You can also stir-fry the stems of the Swiss chard, if you like. Finely chop them and add them to the pan for a pop of color and extra crunch.*

PER SERVING Calories: 353; Total Fat: 21g; Total Carbohydrates: 14g; Sugar: 10g; Fiber: 3g; Protein: 28g; Sodium: 540mg

OPEN-FACED TUNA-AVOCADO SALAD SANDWICHES

SERVES 4   PREP TIME: 10 MINUTES   COOK TIME: 0 MINUTES

CORN FREE
DAIRY FREE
EGG FREE
GLUTEN FREE
NIGHTSHADE FREE
NUT FREE
SOY FREE

I have a secret: you don't need mayonnaise to make a great tuna salad sandwich. If you have nostalgic memories of soggy tuna sandwiches in your lunch bag, get ready to replace them with something completely different. Creamy avocado is the perfect substitute for mayonnaise, with a payload of vitamins, minerals, and healthy fats along for the ride.

3 (6-ounce) cans wild tuna, drained

1 large avocado, halved and pitted

1 celery stalk, finely chopped

½ cup fresh parsley, minced

8 slices gluten-free bread, or Quinoa Flatbread (page 76)

1   In a medium bowl, roughly mash the tuna.

2   Scoop the avocado flesh into the bowl with the tuna. Mash together well.

3   Stir in the celery and parsley.

4   Divide the tuna salad among 4 bread slices. Top each with a second bread slice and serve.

SUBSTITUTION TIP: *If you can tolerate hard-boiled eggs, mashed avocado is also a great alternative to mayonnaise in egg salad sandwiches.*

PER SERVING Calories: 503; Total Fat: 25g; Total Carbohydrates: 31g; Sugar: 1g; Fiber: 7g; Protein: 35g; Sodium: 75mg

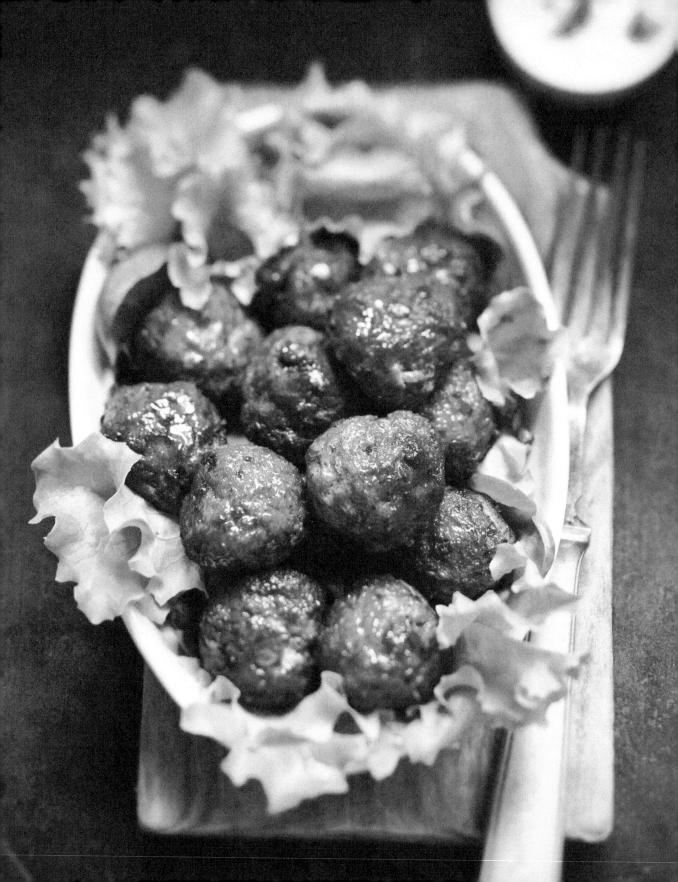

MEAT and POULTRY DISHES

8

BROWN RICE CONGEE

SERVES 6   PREP TIME: 10 MINUTES
COOK TIME: 1 HOUR 30 MINUTES TO 2 HOURS

CORN FREE

DAIRY FREE

EGG FREE

GLUTEN FREE

NIGHTSHADE FREE

NUT FREE

SOY FREE

Congee is an Asian porridge made with rice cooked in lots of water over a long period of time. It's incredibly soothing and comforting, particularly when you're suffering from a cold or stomachache. You can customize congee based on the flavors, meats, and vegetables you like. Experiment by adding leftover cooked meat, fish, scallions, roasted garlic, shredded carrot, bok choy, kale—whatever you're in the mood for.

2½ cups brown rice, rinsed well

7 to 8 cups Basic Chicken Broth (page 93), plus additional as needed

1-inch piece fresh ginger, grated

1 teaspoon salt

3 cups lightly packed spinach leaves

2 tablespoons toasted sesame oil (optional)

1   In a large pot set over high heat, combine the rice, broth, ginger, and salt. Bring to a boil, then reduce the heat to low. Cover and cook for 1½ to 2 hours, stirring occasionally. If the congee becomes too thick, add additional broth.

2   When the congee is cooked, stir in the spinach and let it wilt for about 5 minutes.

3   Drizzle with sesame oil (if using) and serve.

SUBSTITUTION TIP: *Rice is traditionally used for congee, but you can substitute other gluten-free grains. Millet, buckwheat, and quinoa work well, or use a mix of different grains.*

COOKING TIP: *This recipe can also be made in a slow cooker. Combine the rice, ginger, salt, and 6 cups of broth in a slow cooker. Cook on high for 4 hours, or on low for 6 to 8 hours. Add the spinach before serving.*

NOTE *that the Week Three Plan calls for leftovers; double the quantities so you have enough for later in the week.*

PER SERVING Calories: 384; Total Fat: 9g; Total Carbohydrates: 63g; Sugar: 1g; Fiber: 13g; Protein: 13g; Sodium: 1033mg

BUBBIE'S COMFORTING CHICKEN SOUP

SERVES 6   PREP TIME: 20 MINUTES
COOK TIME: 1 HOUR 30 MINUTES TO 2 HOURS

CORN FREE
DAIRY FREE
EGG FREE
GLUTEN FREE
NIGHTSHADE FREE
NUT FREE
SOY FREE
PALEO

"Bubbie" is the Yiddish word for "Grandma," and there were few things I loved more as a child than my own Bubbie's chicken soup dotted with matzo balls, which I would devour by the bowlful. I now know it tasted so good because it was plentiful in fat and salt. This pared-down version of Bubbie's soup uses a shortcut for the broth—you still receive some of the nourishing benefits but without all the fat and salt. Enjoy!

10 bone-in skinless chicken pieces, a mix of legs and thighs (about 3 pounds total)

8 to 10 cups water, divided

1 large onion, washed

4 carrots, peeled and chopped

4 celery stalks, chopped

1 bunch fresh parsley, stemmed and minced

1 teaspoon salt, plus additional as needed

1   In a large pot set over high heat, combine the chicken with 8 cups of water.

2   Add the whole onion to the pot.

3   Bring to a boil. Reduce the heat to medium-low. Cover and cook for 1 hour. If scum rises to the top, skim it off.

4   After 1 hour, remove the onion from the pot. Add the carrots, celery, parsley, and salt. Cover the pot and simmer the soup for 30 minutes more. Add some of the remaining 2 cups of water, as needed.

5   Remove the chicken from the pot. Debone and shred the meat.

6   Return the chicken meat to the pot.

7   Stir, taste, adjust the seasoning if needed, and serve.

INGREDIENT TIP: *If you have extra vegetables, add them to the soup along with the carrots and celery. To boost the anti-inflammatory benefit even further, add some chopped ginger and ground turmeric.*

PER SERVING Calories: 471; Total Fat: 36g; Total Carbohydrates: 7g; Sugar: 3g; Fiber: 2g; Protein: 31g; Sodium: 592mg

BALSAMIC-GLAZED CHICKEN THIGHS with STEAMED CAULIFLOWER

SERVES 4   PREP TIME: 10 MINUTES   COOK TIME: 35 TO 40 MINUTES

CORN FREE
DAIRY FREE
EGG FREE
GLUTEN FREE
NIGHTSHADE FREE
NUT FREE
SOY FREE
PALEO

For a decade I was a vegetarian, and a strict vegan for three of those years. Suddenly, I found myself working as a holistic chef for a family that followed a Paleo diet. My local butcher became my meat guru. He advised that bone-in chicken thighs and legs were the way to go, as they could stand up to lengthy cooking times and still stay tender. They're hands-off to cook and are less expensive than chicken breasts. For this recipe, leave the skin on or take it off; either way, it's delicious.

½ cup balsamic vinegar

¼ cup extra-virgin olive oil

2 tablespoons maple syrup

8 (2- to 3-ounce) bone-in chicken thighs

2 cauliflower heads, broken or cut into florets

Salt, for seasoning

1   In a small bowl, whisk together the balsamic vinegar, olive oil, and maple syrup.

2   In a medium dish, combine the chicken thighs and vinegar-maple mixture. Marinate the chicken for 30 minutes in the refrigerator.

3   Preheat the oven to 350°F.

4   Cover the chicken with aluminum foil and place it in the preheated oven. Bake for 30 to 35 minutes, or until the chicken is cooked through. The internal temperature should read 165°F.

5   If you've left the skin on the chicken, leave the chicken in the oven (uncovered) for an additional 10 minutes to crisp the skin.

6   Fill a large pot with 2 inches of water and insert a steamer basket. Bring to a boil over high heat. Add the cauliflower. Cover and steam for 8 minutes.

7   Serve the chicken with the cauliflower. Drizzle the extra marinade from the casserole dish over the cauliflower, and season with salt, if needed.

MAKE AHEAD TIP: *Marinate the chicken in the sauce in the refrigerator overnight. The extra marinating time will pump up the flavor.*

PER SERVING Calories: 535; Total Fat: 38g; Total Carbohydrates: 14g; Sugar: 9g; Fiber: 3g; Protein: 33g; Sodium: 170mg

TURKEY CHILI

SERVES 6   PREP TIME: 15 MINUTES   COOK TIME: 1 HOUR

CORN FREE
DAIRY FREE
EGG FREE
GLUTEN FREE
NUT FREE
SOY FREE
PALEO

If you're feeding picky eaters, you usually can't go wrong with chili. This filling dish has a simple appeal, and is easy to assemble when you're in a time crunch. If you have prewashed spinach in the refrigerator, throw that in at the end, too. Note that tomatoes are on the acidic side, so if the cans are lined with BPA, the acid will eat at the lining and leach into the tomatoes. Look for BPA-free cans. If that's not an option, choose tomatoes packed in glass.

2 onions, finely diced

8 garlic cloves, minced

2 tablespoons water

1½ pounds ground turkey

6 cups crushed or diced tomatoes

2 tablespoons chili powder, plus additional as needed

1 teaspoon salt, plus additional as needed

1   In a large pot set over medium heat, sauté the onions and garlic with the water for about 5 minutes, or until soft.

2   Add the ground turkey, breaking it up with a spoon, and cook for 5 minutes more.

3   Stir in the tomatoes, chili powder, and salt. Bring to a boil. Reduce the heat to low. Cover and simmer for 45 minutes, stirring occasionally. If the chili gets too dry, add more water.

4   Taste and adjust the seasoning, if necessary.

COOKING TIP: *This recipe can also be made in the slow cooker. Follow steps 1 and 2 then transfer the onions, garlic, and turkey to the slow cooker. You won't need as much liquid, so add only 4 cups of tomatoes and the chili powder. Cook on high for 4 hours, or on low for 6 to 8 hours.*

PER SERVING Calories: 350; Total Fat: 13g; Total Carbohydrates: 26g; Sugar: 16g; Fiber: 10g; Protein: 38g; Sodium: 1016mg

APPLE-TURKEY BURGERS

SERVES 4 TO 6   PREP TIME: 15 MINUTES   COOK TIME: 30 MINUTES

Your family will "gobble" these up and they're practically fool-proof to make. Part of the cooking process is learning to trust your intuition. Get in there with your hands. Does the mixture seem too wet? Add more flour. Too dry? A tablespoon of water. And don't forget the generous pinch of love.

1 red onion, finely chopped

1 apple, washed and grated

1 pound ground turkey

¼ cup chickpea flour, plus additional as needed

½ teaspoon salt

1   Preheat the oven to 350°F.

2   Line a baking sheet with parchment paper.

3   In a large bowl, combine the onion and apple.

4   Add the ground turkey, chickpea flour, and salt. Mix well. If your mixture seems too wet, add another 1 or 2 tablespoons of chickpea flour.

5   Using a ⅓-cup measure, scoop the turkey mixture onto the prepared sheet. Flatten the patties with the bottom of the measure so they are ¾ to 1 inch thick.

6   Place the sheet in the preheated oven and bake for 30 minutes, or until the burgers are cooked through, are opaque in the middle, and the internal temperature reaches 165°F.

SUBSTITUTION TIP: *To make these burgers Paleo, substitute almond flour for the chickpea flour. You can also serve them in lettuce wraps instead of gluten-free buns.*

COOKING TIP: *These burgers can be made on the stove top. In a skillet, heat some coconut oil over medium heat and sauté the patties for 7 to 8 minutes per side, or until cooked through. Be gentle when flipping them.*

PER SERVING Calories: 301; Total Fat: 13g; Total Carbohydrates: 16g; Sugar: 7g; Fiber: 4g; Protein: 34g; Sodium: 417mg

GLAZED CHICKEN with BROCCOLI

SERVES 4   PREP TIME: 15 MINUTES   COOK TIME: 35 MINUTES

If you're tired of the same old chicken, nothing amps up poultry like a sweet honey glaze. The initial sear on the chicken happens on the stove top and then this dish finishes in the oven. So, relax and put your feet up before dinner.

¼ cup coconut oil, divided

1 pound chicken breasts, cut into chunks

¼ cup raw honey

3 broccoli heads, chopped

1 teaspoon salt

2 tablespoons sesame seeds

1   Preheat the oven to 350°F.

2   In a large ovenproof dish or pot set over medium heat, heat 2 tablespoons of coconut oil.

3   Add the chicken. Sauté for 10 minutes.

4   Stir in the honey until well combined. Turn off the heat.

5   Add the broccoli to the pot.

6   Sprinkle with the salt.

7   Cover the pot and place it into the preheated oven. Bake for 20 minutes. Remove the lid and cook for 5 minutes more.

8   Sprinkle with the sesame seeds and serve.

EQUIPMENT TIP: *If you don't have a pot that can transition from stove top to oven, sear the chicken in a sauté pan first and then transfer it to an ovenproof dish before adding the broccoli.*

PER SERVING Calories: 470; Total Fat: 25g; Total Carbohydrates: 28g; Sugar: 20g; Fiber: 4g; Protein: 38g; Sodium: 725mg

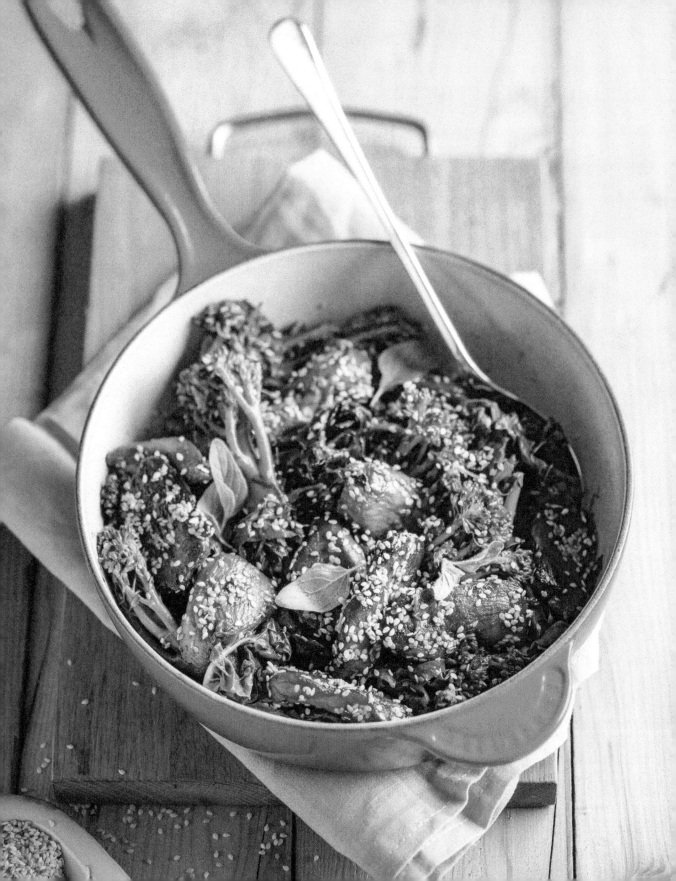

CHICKEN SLIDERS

SERVES 4   PREP TIME: 10 MINUTES   COOK TIME: 30 MINUTES

CORN FREE
DAIRY FREE
EGG FREE
GLUTEN FREE
NIGHTSHADE FREE
NUT FREE
SOY FREE
PALEO

These mini-burgers are fun to serve at a party speared with pickles and tomatoes, but they also make a great meal when paired with roasted vegetables or a salad. Since they're small, these sliders are wonderful for kids, too. No need for burger buns here—enjoy these on their own or wrapped in lettuce if you want a burger covering.

¼ cup quinoa flour, brown rice flour, or chickpea flour

1 pound ground chicken

4 scallions, finely sliced

¾ teaspoon salt

2 to 4 tablespoons coconut oil, divided

1   Cover a large plate with parchment paper.

2   In a medium bowl, mix together the quinoa flour and chicken. In a medium bowl, mix together the quinoa flour and the chicken. Fold in the scallions and add the salt.

3   With wet hands, take about 2 tablespoons of the chicken mixture and roll into a ball. Flatten into a patty and place it on the prepared plate. Repeat with the remaining mixture.

4   In a large sauté pan set over medium heat, heat 2 tablespoons of coconut oil.

5   Add the patties, working in batches, and cook for 8 to10 minutes per side. Add more oil to the pan, if needed, for additional batches. Fully cooked patties should register at least 165°F on a meat thermometer.

6   Serve hot.

COOKING TIP: *If you don't want the trouble of frying, bake these patties instead. Preheat the oven to 375°F. Place the sliders on a parchment-lined baking sheet and bake for 20 to 25 minutes, or until fully cooked.*

PER SERVING Calories: 365; Total Fat: 23g; Total Carbohydrates: 3g; Sugar: 0g; Fiber: 0g; Protein: 37g; Sodium: 538mg

BAKED TURKEY MEATBALLS
with ZUCCHINI NOODLES

SERVES 4   PREP TIME: 15 MINUTES   COOK TIME: 25 MINUTES

CORN FREE
DAIRY FREE
EGG FREE
GLUTEN FREE
NIGHTSHADE FREE
NUT FREE
SOY FREE

It is possible to make great meatballs without eggs and white flour. This recipe calls for lean ground turkey, which is not quite as moist as the darker meat, so the meatballs hold together better. If you can't find lean turkey, add 1 to 2 additional tablespoons of chickpea flour to make up the difference. Chickpea flour lends a savory, nutty flavor, but you can also use brown rice flour or almond flour to make it Paleo.

FOR THE NOODLES

4 zucchini

½ cup extra-virgin olive oil

½ cup fresh basil

FOR THE MEATBALLS

1 pound lean ground turkey

3 tablespoons chickpea flour

1 teaspoon salt

TO MAKE THE NOODLES

1   Using a spiral slicer, spiralize the zucchini into noodles. You can also use a vegetable peeler to slice them into thin strips. Transfer to a large serving bowl.

2   In a blender, blend together the olive oil and basil. Drizzle over the noodles.

TO MAKE THE MEATBALLS

1   Preheat the oven to 350°F.

2   Line a baking sheet with parchment paper.

3   In a medium bowl, mix together the ground turkey, chickpea flour, and salt. »

BAKED TURKEY MEATBALLS WITH ZUCCHINI NOODLES *continued*

4   Using 1 tablespoon for each, roll the mixture into meatballs and place them on the prepared sheet.

5   Place the sheet in the preheated oven and bake for 20 to 25 minutes, or until lightly browned and cooked through.

6   Combine the meatballs with the zucchini noodles and serve.

COOKING TIP: *If you don't like cold zucchini noodles, warm them in a pan for 5 minutes before serving.*

PER SERVING Calories: 444; Total Fat: 34g; Total Carbohydrates: 12g; Sugar: 4g; Fiber: 4g; Protein: 27g; Sodium: 689mg

SLOW-COOKER CHICKEN ALFREDO

SERVES 6   PREP TIME: 20 MINUTES   COOK TIME: 4 TO 8 HOURS

CORN FREE
DAIRY FREE
EGG FREE
GLUTEN FREE
NIGHTSHADE FREE
SOY FREE
PALEO

Seriously, you ask? A dairy-free sauce made with cauliflower that tastes like Alfredo sauce? It's true! I promise you will absolutely love this sauce and want to put it on *everything*—and you can. And, while we tend to think of white foods as lacking in nutrition, there are some exceptions. Cauliflower is one. It's extremely rich in vitamin C, and as a member of the cruciferous family, cauliflower also contains anticancer and anti-inflammatory properties.

FOR THE SAUCE

1 large cauliflower head, broken or cut into florets

Heaping ½ cup cashews, soaked in water for at least 4 hours

1 teaspoon salt

¼ cup water, reserved from cooking the cauliflower

FOR THE CHICKEN

6 (2- to 3-ounce) bone-in skinless chicken thighs

4 cups spinach

TO MAKE THE SAUCE

1   Fill a large pot with 2 inches of water and insert a steamer basket. Bring to a boil over high heat.

2   Add the cauliflower to the steamer basket. Cover and steam for 10 to 12 minutes, or until very tender. Reserve ¼ cup of the cooking liquid.

3   In a colander, drain and rinse the cashews.

4   In a blender, combine the cooked cauliflower, cashews, salt, and ¼ cup of the cauliflower cooking liquid. Blend until smooth and creamy. »

TO MAKE THE CHICKEN

1   Place the chicken thighs in a slow cooker.

2   Pour the sauce over the chicken.

3   Cook on high for 3 to 4 hours, or on low for 7 to 8 hours.

4   Transfer the chicken to a work surface. Remove and discard the bones and gristle. Shred the chicken meat.

5   Return the chicken meat to the cooker.

6   Stir in the spinach. Cook for about 5 minutes, or until the spinach wilts.

MAKE AHEAD TIP: *Cooking the sauce ahead really cuts down on prep time. The sauce will keep in the refrigerator for 3 days, and in the freezer for several months.*

SUBSTITUTION TIP: *For those with nut allergies, use ¾ cup of sunflower seeds instead of cashews. And if you've forgotten to soak the cashews, ½ cup of cashew butter will also work.*

NOTE *that the Week Two Plan calls for leftovers; double the quantities so you have enough for later in the week.*

PER SERVING Calories: 286; Total Fat: 18g; Total Carbohydrates: 12g; Sugar: 4g; Fiber: 4g; Protein: 27g; Sodium: 511mg

LAMB-STUFFED PEPPERS

SERVES 6 PREP TIME: 20 MINUTES COOK TIME: 1 HOUR

CORN FREE
DAIRY FREE
EGG FREE
GLUTEN FREE
NUT FREE
SOY FREE
PALEO

Stuffed peppers make a delightful meal—satisfying and delicious in a neat little package. The lovely thing about stuffed peppers is you can use a multitude of ingredients for the filling. So, if you don't like lamb, swap in other ground meats like beef, chicken, or turkey. Create a vegetarian version using cooked quinoa and lentils as a fantastic alternative.

1 onion, finely diced

2 tablespoons water, plus additional for cooking

1½ pounds ground lamb

1 cup grated zucchini (about 1 zucchini)

¼ cup fresh basil, minced

1 teaspoon salt

6 bell peppers, any color, seeded, ribbed, tops removed and reserved

1   Preheat the oven to 350°F.

2   In a large pan set over medium heat, sauté the onion in the water for about 5 minutes, or until soft.

3   Add the ground lamb and zucchini. Cook for 10 minutes, breaking up the meat with a spoon.

4   Stir in the basil and salt. Remove from the heat.

5   Fill a casserole dish with 1½ inches of water.

6   Stuff each pepper with an equal amount of the lamb mixture and place them into the dish. Cap each pepper with its reserved top.

7   Place the dish in the preheated oven and bake for 45 to 50 minutes.

SUBSTITUTION TIP: *For a nightshade-free option, stuff the mixture into acorn squash instead.*

PER SERVING Calories: 258; Total Fat: 9g; Total Carbohydrates: 10g; Sugar: 6g; Fiber: 3g; Protein: 34g; Sodium: 481mg

HERBED LAMB-ZUCCHINI BOATS

SERVES 6   PREP TIME: 15 MINUTES   COOK TIME: 40 MINUTES

Many herbs are delicate, tender, and easily bruised. Not rosemary. It's also filled with calcium and iron, and contains compounds that reduce inflammation, help with digestion, and enhance memory. Rosemary has a fragrant, robust flavor that isn't for everyone, so adjust the amount to suit your tastes.

6 zucchini, ends trimmed, halved lengthwise

1 onion, finely diced

2 tablespoons water

1 pound ground lamb

1 to 2 tablespoons fresh rosemary, minced

½ teaspoon salt

1   Preheat the oven to 350°F.

2   Line a baking sheet with parchment paper.

3   With a small spoon, gently hollow out about 1 inch of space along the length of the inside of the zucchini halves.

4   In a large pan set over medium heat, sauté the onion in the water for about 5 minutes, or until soft.

5   Add the ground lamb, rosemary, and salt. Cook for 10 minutes, breaking up the lamb with a spoon. Remove from the heat.

6   Place the zucchini on the prepared sheet, hollow-side up.

7   Fill each zucchini with equal amounts of the lamb mixture.

8   Place the sheet in the preheated oven and bake for 25 minutes, or until the lamb is fully cooked and the zucchini are tender.

COOKING TIP: *Zucchini boats are great vehicles for all sorts of flavors. They make great pizza "crusts": Simply fill with tomato sauce, and pile on your favorite toppings.*

PER SERVING Calories: 183; Total Fat: 6g; Total Carbohydrates: 9g; Sugar: 4g; Fiber: 3g; Protein: 24g; Sodium: 272mg

POACHED CHICKEN WRAPS

SERVES 4 TO 6   PREP TIME: 30 MINUTES   COOK TIME: 15 MINUTES

This is a meat-based version of Vegetable Spring Roll Wraps (page 107). Poaching chicken is a simple and basic cooking method, and here, it's stripped down further by cooking in water only. When paired with fresh vegetables and herbs, these wraps make for a light and refreshing meal.

2 cups water, plus additional for soaking the wrappers

2 (4-ounce) boneless skinless chicken breasts

10 rice paper wrappers

1 small head romaine lettuce, sliced thin

2 cups lightly packed spinach, sliced thin

½ cup fresh dill, minced

1   In a shallow pan set over high heat, bring the water to a boil. Reduce the heat to medium. Add the chicken breasts. Cover and cook for 15 minutes, or until the chicken is cooked through and the internal temperature is at least 165°F. Remove the chicken from the pot, let it cool, and slice it thinly.

2   Place a cutting board on a flat surface with the fillings in front of you.

3   Fill a large, shallow bowl with warm water. The water should be hot enough to cook the wrappers but warm enough so you can touch it comfortably.

4   Soak one rice paper wrapper in the water, and place it on the cutting board.

5   Place ½ cup of romaine, ¼ cup of spinach, 1 teaspoon of dill, and a few chicken slices in the middle of the wrapper. »

6   Fold the sides in over the fillings. Then, starting at the bottom (the end closest to you), tightly roll up the wrapper burrito-style.

7   Repeat with the remaining wrappers, chicken, and vegetables.

MAKE AHEAD TIP: *Poach, cool, and slice the chicken ahead of time to reduce assembly time later. Keep the chicken refrigerated in a sealed container for 3 to 4 days before using.*

If you aren't serving these right away, the rice paper wrappers will dry out (even if the time between preparing and serving is only an hour). To prevent this, dampen a paper towel or cloth napkin and cover the wraps to keep them moist.

PER SERVING Calories: 255; Total Fat: 5g; Total Carbohydrates: 32g; Sugar: 2g; Fiber: 2g; Protein: 20g; Sodium: 188mg

BRAISED TURKEY LEGS
with WILTED GREENS

SERVES 6   PREP TIME: 15 MINUTES   COOK TIME: 1 HOUR 20 MINUTES

CORN FREE
DAIRY FREE
EGG FREE
GLUTEN FREE
NIGHTSHADE FREE
NUT FREE
SOY FREE
PALEO

This recipe has all the comfort of a turkey dinner—without having to defrost, clean, truss, bake, and baste a whole turkey for hours on end. The result is a simple meal that you can enjoy any day of the week, or any time of the year—you don't even need to turn on the oven.

3 (1½- to 2-pound) turkey legs

¾ teaspoon salt

3 tablespoons coconut oil

1 onion, minced

4 garlic cloves, minced

5 cups water

6 cups lightly packed kale, thoroughly washed and chopped

1   Pat the turkey legs dry and sprinkle with the salt.

2   Add the coconut oil to a large pot set over medium-high heat.

3   Add the turkey legs and sear for about 5 minutes per side. You may need to do this in batches, depending on the size of your pot. Transfer the turkey to a plate and set aside.

4   Add the onion and garlic to the pot. Sauté for about 5 minutes, or until soft.

5   Return the turkey to the pot and add the water. Bring to a boil. Reduce the heat to low. Cover and simmer for 1 hour, or until the meat is tender and starting to fall off the bone.

6   Scatter the kale over the turkey. Stir and cook for about 5 minutes, or until the kale wilts.

SUBSTITUTION TIP: *If you can't find whole turkey legs, use 6 to 8 turkey thighs instead.*

PER SERVING Calories: 731; Total Fat: 37g; Total Carbohydrates: 9g; Sugar: 1g; Fiber: 1g; Protein: 87g; Sodium: 554mg

SESAME CHICKEN STIR-FRY

SERVES 6   PREP TIME: 15 MINUTES   COOK TIME: 25 MINUTES

CORN FREE
DAIRY FREE
EGG FREE
GLUTEN FREE
NIGHTSHADE FREE
NUT FREE
SOY FREE
PALEO

Stir-fries are handy meals when you're short on time, ingredients, and patience. This stir-fry relies heavily on nutty sesame flavor, so it's for big sesame lovers. There is a double dose of calcium here from the tahini and the kale, making it a great option if you're looking to build or maintain bone health. As with all stir-fries, this one welcomes any extra bits in your refrigerator looking for a repurpose.

¾ cup warm water

½ cup tahini

¼ cup plus 2 tablespoons toasted sesame oil, divided

2 garlic cloves, minced

½ teaspoon salt

1 pound boneless skinless chicken breasts, cut into ½-inch cubes

6 cups lightly packed kale, thoroughly washed and chopped

1   In a medium bowl, whisk together the warm water, tahini, ¼ cup of sesame oil, garlic, and salt.

2   In a large pan set over medium heat, heat the remaining 2 table-spoons of sesame oil.

3   Add the chicken and cook for 8 to 10 minutes, stirring.

4   Stir in the tahini-sesame sauce, mixing well to coat the chicken. Cook for 6 to 8 minutes more.

5   One handful at a time, add the kale. When the first handful wilts, add the next. Continue until all the kale has been added. Serve hot.

SUBSTITUTION TIP: *Boneless skinless chicken thighs can also be used in this recipe.*

PER SERVING Calories: 417; Total Fat: 30g; Total Carbohydrates: 12g; Sugar: 0g; Fiber: 3g; Protein: 27g; Sodium: 311mg

COCONUT CHICKEN CURRY

SERVES 6   PREP TIME: 8 MINUTES   COOK TIME: 35 MINUTES

This five-ingredient curry is not authentic in the least, but it is quick, easy, and tasty. Most of the curry-like flavor stems from the curry powder, which you can adjust to suit your taste. Since curry mixes often contain chili powder, there's a chile-free alternative in the recipe notes below. This is also a great option for those who can't tolerate, or just dislike, spicy food.

3 cups coconut milk

2 cups water

1 to 2 tablespoons curry powder

2 pounds boneless skinless chicken thighs, cut into cubes

1 teaspoon salt

3 bunches Swiss chard, washed, stemmed, and roughly chopped

1   In a large pot, combine the coconut milk, water, curry powder, chicken, and salt. Bring to a boil over high heat. Reduce the heat to low. Cover and simmer for 30 minutes.

2   Add the Swiss chard to the pot. Cook for 5 minutes, or until the chard wilts.

SUBSTITUTION TIP: *To make this without nightshades, make your own quick, chile-free version of curry powder. In a small bowl, whisk together 2 teaspoons of ground cumin, 1 teaspoon of ground coriander, 1 teaspoon of ground ginger, and ½ teaspoon of ground turmeric. Add the spices to the curry, taste, and adjust as needed.*

NOTE *that the Week Two Plan calls for leftovers; double the quantities so you have enough for later in the week.*

PER SERVING Calories: 581; Total Fat: 40g; Total Carbohydrates: 10g; Sugar: 5g; Fiber: 4g; Protein: 48g; Sodium: 652mg

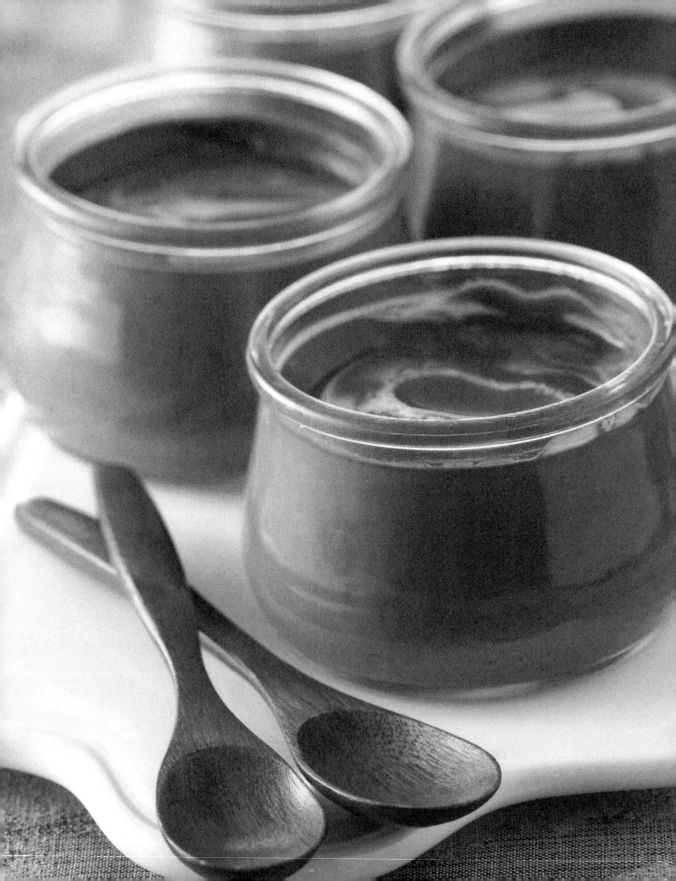

DESSERTS

9

GRAIN-FREE FRUIT CRISP

SERVES 4 TO 6   PREP TIME: 5 MINUTES   COOK TIME: 30 TO 35 MINUTES

This fruit crisp recipe is incredibly versatile. Use a single type of fruit, or a combination of many. And it's a great use for any bruised fruit past its prime. Basically any fruit works—berries, plums, cherries, apples, peaches, nectarines, pears, apricots, mango, pineapple, you name it. I like to make fruit crisps as seasonal as possible, relying on what I find at local markets. With antioxidant-rich fruit, the protein-packed sunflower seeds, and the healthy fats from the coconut products, this is a healthy, guilt-free dessert. I often eat leftovers for breakfast, either alone or dolloped with coconut yogurt.

3 cups mixed fresh berries (raspberries, blueberries, blackberries, etc.)

½ cup sunflower seeds

¾ cup unsweetened shredded coconut

¼ cup coconut sugar

¼ cup coconut oil

1   Preheat the oven to 350°F.

2   In a 9-by-9-inch baking dish, combine the fruit.

3   In a small bowl, mix together the sunflower seeds, shredded coconut, and coconut sugar.

4   Stir in the coconut oil and incorporate it throughout. It's easier if you use your hands.

5   Crumble the topping over the fruit.

6   Place the dish in the preheated oven and bake for 30 to 35 minutes, or until the topping is golden and the fruit is bubbling.

SUBSTITUTION TIP: *You can use any nut or seed in the topping. If it's a larger nut, like almonds, pecans, or walnuts, give them a rough chop before mixing with the rest of the topping ingredients.*

PER SERVING Calories: 379; Total Fat: 29g; Total Carbohydrates: 29g; Sugar: 18g; Fiber: 10g; Protein: 4g; Sodium: 9mg

CHOCOLATE-AVOCADO PUDDING

SERVES 4   PREP TIME: 10 MINUTES   COOK TIME: 0 MINUTES

CORN FREE
DAIRY FREE
EGG FREE
GLUTEN FREE
NIGHTSHADE FREE
NUT FREE
SOY FREE
PALEO
VEGAN

Dates are an incredibly nutritious natural sweetener. They're rich in fiber, B vitamins, and important minerals like calcium, iron, magnesium, and potassium. Amazing, no? They make a great snack when stuffed with nut or seed butter, and can amp up the nutrient factor in a wide variety of desserts. I use soft, caramel-like Medjool dates, but try any you like. If your dates are a little dry, soak them in warm water for 5 minutes before blending the pudding.

12 Medjool dates, pitted

2 avocados, halved and pitted

½ cup cacao powder

1 cup coconut milk, divided

1   In a food processor, combine the dates, avocado flesh, cacao powder, and ¾ cup of coconut milk. Blend until smooth. If the pudding is too thick, add the remaining ¼ cup of coconut milk and blend well.

2   Refrigerate for 1 hour before serving.

INGREDIENT TIP: *To enhance the flavor, add vanilla extract, peppermint extract, ground cinnamon, ground ginger, or even a pinch of ground turmeric.*

PER SERVING Calories: 488; Total Fat: 36g; Total Carbohydrates: 48g; Sugar: 28g; Fiber: 14g; Protein: 6g; Sodium: 15mg

STRAWBERRY JAM THUMBPRINT COOKIES

SERVES 4 TO 6   PREP TIME: 15 MINUTES   COOK TIME: 15 MINUTES

CORN FREE
DAIRY FREE
EGG FREE
GLUTEN FREE
NIGHTSHADE FREE
NUT FREE
SOY FREE
PALEO
VEGAN

Using only four ingredients and a half-hour of your time, you can have a delicious batch of cookies ready to be devoured. There really is no excuse for *not* making these. Enjoy them for dessert or as a quick, energy-boosting snack. With the power pack of vitamin E in the sunflower seeds and the copious amounts of vitamin C in the jam, it's like munching on a mouthful of antioxidants.

1½ cups sunflower seeds

3 tablespoons coconut oil

¼ cup maple syrup

½ cup strawberry jam, divided

1   Preheat the oven to 350°F.

2   Line a baking sheet with parchment paper.

3   In a blender, food processor, or spice grinder, process the sunflower seeds into a fine meal. Transfer to a large bowl.

4   Add the coconut oil, mashing it into the sunflower meal with a spoon as if you are crumbling butter into flour. Stir in the maple syrup. Mix well.

5   Using a tablespoon measure, scoop the dough onto the prepared sheet, making 12 cookies. Gently press down on the cookies with the back of a wet spoon to flatten them.

6   With your thumb, make imprints in the center of each cookie. Fill each depression with 2 teaspoons of strawberry jam.

7   Place the sheet in the preheated oven and bake for 12 to 14 minutes.

8   Cool before eating.

SUBSTITUTION TIP: *You can use any type of jam in these cookies. They're also fun to eat when you fill them with nut butter or dairy-free dark chocolate chips.*

PER SERVING Calories: 392; Total Fat: 19g; Total Carbohydrates: 54g; Sugar: 12g; Fiber: 2g; Protein: 4g; Sodium: 3mg

SEEDY COOKIE DOUGH BITES

SERVES 4 TO 6   PREP TIME: 12 MINUTES   COOK TIME: 0 MINUTES

CORN FREE
DAIRY FREE
EGG FREE
GLUTEN FREE
NIGHTSHADE FREE
NUT FREE
SOY FREE
VEGAN

This is the perfect no-bake, no-hassle recipe for parties or pot-lucks. While you may be tempted to eat them all yourself, they're so nutritionally dense that you don't need many to feel satisfied. If you're in the mood to be extra decadent, melt ½ cup of dark chocolate and use it to give the bites an elegant drizzle, or coat them entirely with a chocolate shell.

⅔ cup pumpkin seeds

⅔ cup sunflower seeds

⅔ cup gluten-free rolled oats

¼ cup maple syrup

1 teaspoon vanilla extract

¼ cup cacao nibs, or dairy-free chocolate chips

1   Line a large plate with parchment paper.

2   In a food processor, combine the pumpkin seeds, sunflower seeds, and oats. Process into a fine meal.

3   Add the maple syrup and vanilla. Blend until combined.

4   Add the cacao nibs and pulse together.

5   Using a 1-tablespoon measure, roll 12-16 cookie balls with your hands. Place them on the prepared plate.

6   Freeze the dough balls for 30 minutes to firm. Transfer to a sealed container. Refrigerate.

INGREDIENT TIP: *Because the oils in all nuts and seeds are delicate, I store them in the refrigerator or freezer so they don't become rancid.*

PER SERVING Calories: 345; Total Fat: 19g; Total Carbohydrates: 36g; Sugar: 12g; Fiber: 6g; Protein: 12g; Sodium: 7mg

COCONUT-BLUEBERRY POPSICLES

SERVES 6   PREP TIME: 15 MINUTES   COOK TIME: 0 MINUTES

Ice pops are one of those treats that many people tend to buy, but they are really very simple to make at home—and homemade versions don't have the artificial colors and flavors found in the commercial versions. Ice pop molds are inexpensive and a great investment, but you can also make ice pops with paper cups and popsicle sticks. Making these is a great cooking activity for children—and a great way to get them to eat more fruit!

1 cup fresh blueberries

1½ cups coconut milk

¼ cup maple syrup

¼ teaspoon cinnamon

⅛ teaspoon salt

1   In a small bowl, roughly mash the blueberries.

2   Divide the blueberry mixture among 6 ice pop molds.

3   In a medium bowl, mix together the coconut milk, maple syrup, cinnamon, and salt.

4   Pour the coconut milk mixture into the ice pop molds over the blueberries.

5   Freeze for at least 2 hours, or until solid.

INGREDIENT TIP: *In this recipe, I like to mash the blueberries so they still have a little texture. If you prefer them completely smooth, purée in a blender before adding them to the molds.*

SUBSTITUTION TIP: *This recipe works with a variety of fruit. If you aren't in the mood for berries, use peaches, apricots, nectarines, plums, figs, cherries, or kiwi. You can also add some chopped dark chocolate or dark chocolate chips for extra flavor and nutrition.*

PER SERVING Calories: 186; Total Fat: 14g; Total Carbohydrates: 16g; Sugar: 12g; Fiber: 2g; Protein: 2g; Sodium: 37mg

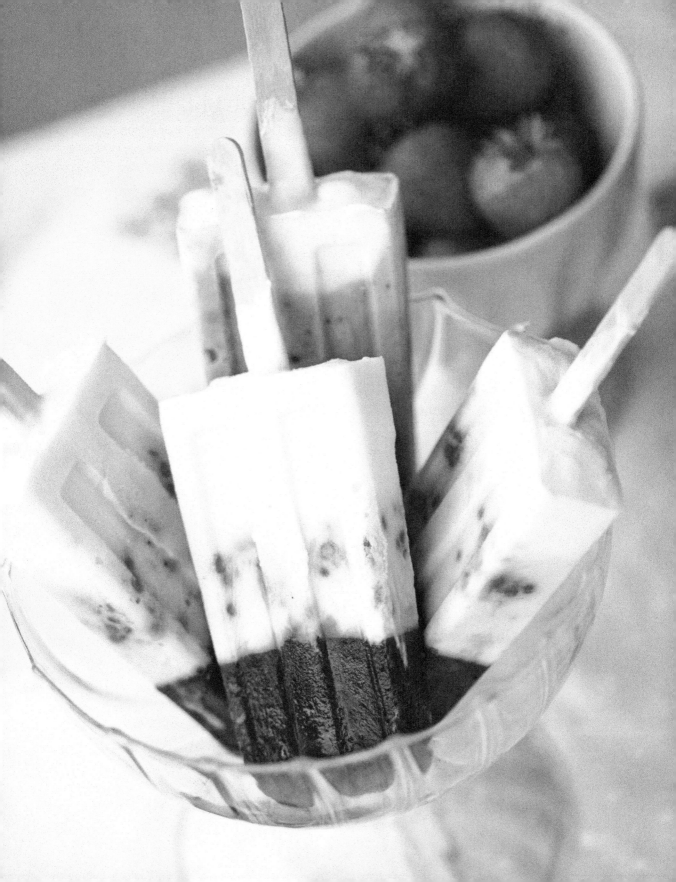

YOUR NEW FAVORITE VANILLA ICE CREAM

SERVES 6 TO 8   PREP TIME: 10 MINUTES   COOK TIME: 0 MINUTES

Homemade ice cream isn't difficult or time consuming, and you can create whatever flavor you want. You don't even need an ice cream maker. The secret to creamy, luxurious dairy-free ice cream is fat, particularly if you don't have an ice cream machine. So don't skimp on the coconut milk: choose a full-fat version, or use coconut cream concentrate if you can find it, as it's even thicker than the milk. Eat this ice cream as is, or jazz it up with dairy-free chocolate chips, nuts, fresh fruit, cookie chunks, or cacao powder.

3 cups full-fat coconut milk

⅓ cup maple syrup

2 teaspoons vanilla extract, or ½ teaspoon vanilla powder

¼ teaspoon salt

1   In a large bowl, whisk together the coconut milk, maple syrup, vanilla, and salt. Alternately, use a blender to combine.

2   If using an ice cream maker, freeze according to the manufacturer's instructions. Transfer the ice cream to a sealed container and store in the freezer.

3   If not using an ice cream maker, pour the mixture into a container and freeze. You can also freeze some of the mixture in ice cube trays to add to smoothies.

INGREDIENT TIP: *Vanilla powder is made from whole vanilla beans that have been dried and ground. It's an expensive ingredient, but a little goes a long way—you don't have to use as much as extract to achieve a wonderful vanilla flavor. Since I discovered vanilla powder, I've found it hard to go back to extract.*

PER SERVING Calories: 296; Total Fat: 24g; Total Carbohydrates: 18g; Sugar: 14g; Fiber: 0g; Protein: 2g; Sodium: 129mg

COCONUT-CHOCOLATE CLUMPS

MAKES 12 TO 16 PIECES   PREP TIME: 10 MINUTES   COOK TIME: 5 MINUTES

CORN FREE
DAIRY FREE
EGG FREE
GLUTEN FREE
NIGHTSHADE FREE
NUT FREE
SOY FREE
PALEO
VEGAN

Chocolate not only tastes good but also has an abundance of antioxidants, magnesium, and iron, and can be a healthy choice depending on the source. It's raw chocolate—or cacao—that offers all the benefits. Making your own chocolate is incredibly satisfying, not to mention simple. If you don't have candy molds, make chocolate bark instead: Line a loaf pan with parchment paper and pour the chocolate mixture into it. Once solid, break it into pieces.

¼ cup cacao powder

¼ cup maple syrup

3 tablespoons coconut oil

1 tablespoon cacao butter

½ cup unsweetened shredded coconut

Pinch salt

1   Create a makeshift double boiler: Fill a small pot with a few inches of water and place a metal bowl on top of the pot. Bring the water to a boil.

2   Put the cacao powder, maple syrup, coconut oil, and cacao butter into the bowl. Use oven mitts when handling the bowl, as it will be hot!

3   Stir the chocolate mixture until it melts, about 5 minutes.

4   With the mitts, remove the bowl from the top of the pot. Stir in the shredded coconut.

5   Pour the chocolate mixture into candy molds.

6   Refrigerate or freeze until set.

SUBSTITUTION TIP: *Cacao butter is made from the fat extracted from the cacao bean. It lends additional chocolate-y texture and mouthfeel. If you can't find it, use one extra tablespoon of coconut oil.*

PER SERVING Calories: 91; Total Fat: 8g; Total Carbohydrates: 6g; Sugar: 4g; Fiber: 1g; Protein: 1g; Sodium: 14mg

ALMOND BUTTER FREEZER FUDGE

SERVES 6 TO 8   PREP TIME: 5 MINUTES   COOK TIME: 5 MINUTES

CORN FREE
DAIRY FREE
EGG FREE
GLUTEN FREE
NIGHTSHADE FREE
SOY FREE
PALEO
VEGAN

Traditional fudge is loaded with sugar and butter, but you won't find any of those inflammatory ingredients here. Instead, treat yourself with satiating, healthy fats; protein; and a touch of sweetness. A small square of this fudge is a great way to finish a meal, but given its health-building benefits, it can also be a nice snack or easy-to-digest pre-workout boost.

⅓ cup coconut oil

¾ cup almond butter

¼ cup maple syrup

¼ teaspoon salt

1   Line a loaf pan with parchment paper.

2   In a small pot set over low heat, combine the coconut oil, almond butter, maple syrup, and salt. Warm gently for about 5 minutes, or until everything is incorporated.

3   Pour the fudge into the prepared pan, smoothing it evenly.

4   Refrigerate for 1 hour.

5   Slice the fudge into 12–16 squares.

6   Store in a sealed container in the freezer.

SUBSTITUTION TIP: *For a nut-free version, use tahini or sunflower seed butter in place of the almond butter.*

PER SERVING Calories: 350; Total Fat: 31g; Total Carbohydrates: 14g; Sugar: 8g; Fiber: 1g; Protein: 7g; Sodium: 98mg

CHOCOLATE FONDUE

SERVES 4 TO 6   PREP TIME: 10 MINUTES   COOK TIME: 5 MINUTES

CORN FREE
DAIRY FREE
EGG FREE
GLUTEN FREE
NIGHTSHADE FREE
NUT FREE
SOY FREE
PALEO
VEGAN

It's a fact: Everything tastes better when it's been dipped in chocolate. This effortless and quick recipe will impress your guests or your family, and is fun to eat—though the melted chocolate can get messy, so be prepared. No fancy fondue pot is needed here; any bowl will do. Fruit is a fantastic choice for dipping, but you can use gluten-free cookies or gluten-free cake, too. If you're entertaining a crowd, this recipe can easily be doubled or tripled.

½ cup cacao powder

¼ cup coconut oil

¼ cup maple syrup, or raw honey

4 cups fresh fruit for dipping (berries, bananas, pitted cherries, pineapple, etc.), sliced or cut into bite-size pieces

1   Create a makeshift double boiler: Fill a small pot with a few inches of water and place a metal bowl on top of the pot. Bring the water to a boil.

2   Put the cacao powder, coconut oil, and maple syrup into the bowl. Use oven mitts when handling the bowl, as it will be hot!

3   Stir the chocolate mixture until it melts, about 5 minutes. Transfer to a serving bowl or individual bowls for dipping.

SUBSTITUTION TIP: *If you enjoy the taste of carob, use it instead of cacao powder. Carob has a similar nutrient profile to cacao, including antioxidants, calcium, iron, and fiber, but with no caffeine.*

PER SERVING Calories: 452; Total Fat: 16g; Total Carbohydrates: 83g; Sugar: 17g; Fiber: 8g; Protein: 6g; Sodium: 8mg

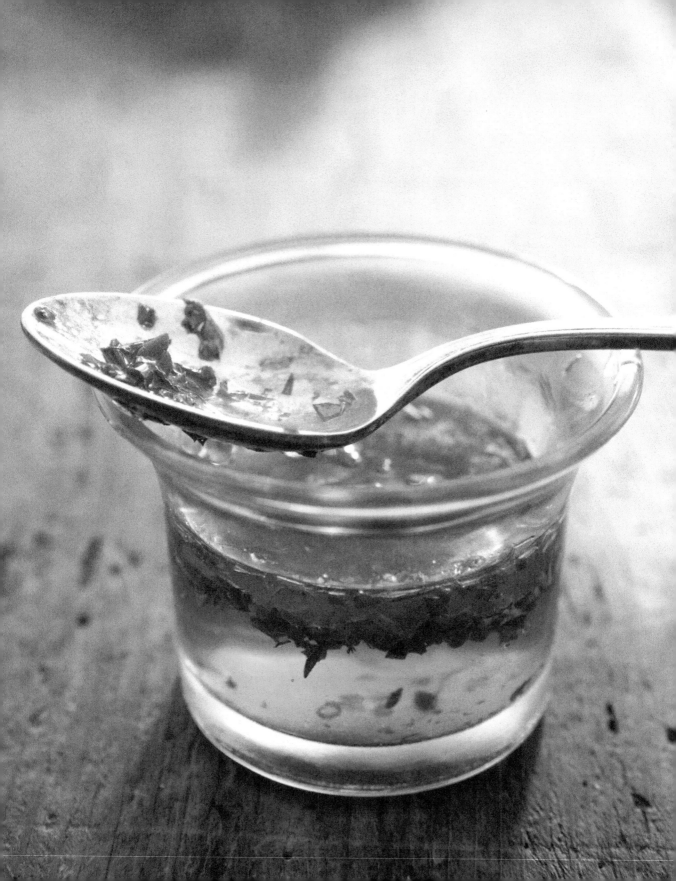

SAUCES, CONDIMENTS, and DRESSINGS 10

ADDICTIVE MULTI-PURPOSE CREAM SAUCE

MAKES 3½ CUPS   PREP TIME: 10 MINUTES   COOK TIME: 12 MINUTES

CORN FREE
DAIRY FREE
EGG FREE
GLUTEN FREE
NIGHTSHADE FREE
SOY FREE
PALEO
VEGAN

I named this recipe for a reason: It's awesome and addictive. I keep a jar on hand in the freezer so I'll always have a tasty meal-booster in case of emergency. It works with everything, whether hot or cold—on cooked vegetables, meat, fish, pasta, grains, salad, and bread. It almost has a cheesy flavor, even though it's dairy free. A favorite combination is this sauce with pasta, cooked salmon, and kale. Throw it in the oven and it will come out tasting like a baked mac and cheese. Try it yourself and see!

3 cups cubed butternut squash

½ cup cashews, soaked in water for at least 4 hours, drained

½ cup water, plus additional for cooking and thinning

1 teaspoon salt, plus additional as needed

1   Fill a large pot with 2 inches of water and insert a steamer basket. Bring to a boil over high heat.

2   Add the butternut squash to the basket. Cover and steam for 10 to 12 minutes, or until tender.

3   Remove from the heat and cool slightly.

4   Transfer the squash to a blender. Add the cashews, ½ cup of water, and salt. Blend until smooth and creamy. Depending on the consistency, add more water to thin if necessary.

5   Taste, and adjust the seasoning if necessary.

SUBSTITUTION TIP: *Any variety of squash will work in this recipe: butternut, delicata, acorn, pumpkin, and Hubbard are just a few options. I've also made it with sweet potatoes with great success. If nut allergies are an issue, use soaked sunflower seeds, or ½ cup of tahini instead of the cashews.*

PER SERVING (½ cup) Calories: 73; Total Fat: 5g; Total Carbohydrates: 8g; Sugar: 1g; Fiber: 1g; Protein: 2g; Sodium: 335mg

GARLIC-TAHINI SAUCE

MAKES 1 CUP   PREP TIME: 10 MINUTES   COOK TIME: 0 MINUTES

CORN FREE
DAIRY FREE
EGG FREE
GLUTEN FREE
NIGHTSHADE FREE
NUT FREE
SOY FREE
PALEO
VEGAN

There is a reason garlic is affectionately called "the stinking rose." It's strong, and packed with so many important anti-inflammatory, antibacterial, and anticancer compounds. Garlic is far more potent raw than cooked, which is why there is just one clove in this sauce. If you love the taste of raw garlic, add another clove or two! Just don't expect to be kissed.

½ cup tahini

1 garlic clove, minced

Juice of 1 lemon

Zest of 1 lemon

½ teaspoon salt, plus additional as needed

½ cup warm water, plus additional as needed

1   In a small bowl, stir together the tahini and garlic.

2   Add the lemon juice, lemon zest, and salt. Stir well.

3   Whisk in ½ cup of warm water, until well mixed and creamy. Add more water if the sauce is too thick.

4   Taste, and adjust the seasoning if necessary.

5   Refrigerate in a sealed container.

PREPARATION TIP: *Tahini condenses a lot in the refrigerator. If you make this sauce ahead of time, it will get ultra-thick when cooled. When you're ready to use it, add a few tablespoons of hot water to achieve a runnier consistency.*

PER SERVING (¼ cup) Calories: 180; Total Fat: 16g; Total Carbohydrates: 7g; Sugar: 0g; Fiber: 3g; Protein: 5g; Sodium: 325mg

RED WINE and PARSLEY VINAIGRETTE

MAKES ABOUT ½ CUP   PREP TIME: 5 MINUTES   COOK TIME: 0 MINUTES

CORN FREE
DAIRY FREE
EGG FREE
GLUTEN FREE
NIGHTSHADE FREE
NUT FREE
SOY FREE
PALEO
VEGAN

Parsley deserves star treatment, and shouldn't be relegated to the side of the plate as a garnish. It's an incredibly rich source of iron, as well as the anti-inflammatory vitamins A, C, and K. If you're looking for even more reasons to love parsley, its high levels of antioxidants—particularly *glutathione*, an antioxidant that is particularly important because it works within cells—help protect against free-radical damage and assist with ousting harmful chemicals from the body.

⅓ cup extra-virgin olive oil

3 tablespoons red wine vinegar

1 garlic clove, minced

½ cup lightly packed fresh parsley, finely chopped

¼ teaspoon salt, plus additional as needed

1   In a small jar, combine the olive oil, red wine vinegar, garlic, parsley, and salt. Seal the jar and shake until mixed.

2   Taste, and adjust the seasoning if necessary.

3   Refrigerate.

SUBSTITUTION TIP: *If you don't like red wine vinegar, or can't find it, substitute rice wine vinegar or apple cider vinegar.*

PER SERVING (1 tablespoon) Calories: 93; Total Fat: 11g; Total Carbohydrates: 0g; Sugar: 0g; Fiber: 0g; Protein: 0g; Sodium: 76mg

ROASTED FENNEL and SUNFLOWER SEED PESTO

MAKES 2 CUPS   PREP TIME: 15 MINUTES   COOK TIME: 30 MINUTES

CORN FREE
DAIRY FREE
EGG FREE
GLUTEN FREE
NIGHTSHADE FREE
NUT FREE
SOY FREE
PALEO
VEGAN

This recipe is a riff on traditional pesto, which is usually made with basil, pine nuts, and Parmesan cheese. Fennel garners its digestive powers from a volatile oil called *anethole*. Anethole helps reduce indigestion and gas, and moves food through the digestive tract. Roasting gives the fennel a sweeter, caramelized flavor, which is complemented here by toasty garlic and bright lemon.

2 fennel bulbs

8 garlic cloves, peeled

2 tablespoons extra-virgin olive oil, plus additional as needed

¾ cup sunflower seeds

¼ cup freshly squeezed lemon juice

½ teaspoon sea salt, plus additional as needed

1   Preheat the oven to 350°F.

2   Trim the fronds from the fennel bulbs and set aside. Cut off the stalks and save them for another use, such as Basic Chicken Broth (page 93). Halve the fennel bulbs, removing and discarding the core. Chop the fennel roughly.

3   In a large roasting pan, combine the chopped fennel and garlic.

4   Drizzle with the olive oil and toss to coat.

5   Place the pan in the preheated oven and roast for 30 minutes, stirring halfway through. Remove the pan from the oven and cool.

6   In a food processor, grind the sunflower seeds into a rough meal. »

7   Add the roasted fennel and garlic, along with the lemon juice and sea salt. Process until everything comes together. If the pesto is dry, add an additional 1 or 2 tablespoons of olive oil, or water.

8   Roughly chop a handful of the reserved fennel fronds. Add them to the pesto. Pulse until combined. Taste, and adjust the seasoning if necessary.

INGREDIENT TIP: *If you're not making broth anytime in the near future, freeze the fennel stalks in a freezer-safe bag or sealed container. You'll have it when you need it to give your broth a boost of digestive power.*

PER SERVING (¼ cup) Calories: 80; Total Fat: 6g; Total Carbohydrates: 6g; Sugar: 0g; Fiber: 2g; Protein: 2g; Sodium: 150mg

TOASTED COCONUT SUNBUTTER

MAKES 1½ CUPS   PREP TIME: 10 MINUTES   COOK TIME: 6 TO 8 MINUTES

CORN FREE
DAIRY FREE
EGG FREE
GLUTEN FREE
NIGHTSHADE FREE
NUT FREE
SOY FREE
PALEO
VEGAN

For those with nut allergies, toasted sunflower seed butter (or sun-butter) is a versatile lifesaver. It's earthy and nutty, and has a peanut butter–like flavor. When combined with coconut, you end up with a delicious cross between seed butter and coconut butter. Spread this on toast, spoon it over oatmeal, cereal, or fruit, or add it to smoothies. You can also use it in savory dishes to add thickness and depth, as a marinade for chicken, or to thicken soups and stews.

1½ cups sunflower seeds

⅛ teaspoon salt

1½ cups large-flake unsweetened coconut

1   Preheat the oven to 350°F.

2   On a baking sheet, spread the sunflower seeds and coconut.

3   Place the sheet in the preheated oven and bake for 6 to 8 minutes. Keep a close watch, as the seeds and coconut can burn quickly.

4   Remove from the oven and cool.

5   In a food processor, combine the seeds, coconut, and salt. Blend until smooth and creamy, scraping down the sides as needed.

6   Pour into a sealable jar.

STORAGE TIP: *Coconut products firm up in cold temperatures. Store this in the refrigerator for a thick nut butter, or keep it in the pantry for a runnier texture.*

PER SERVING (1 tablespoon) Calories: 66; Total Fat: 7g; Total Carbohydrates: 3g; Sugar: 1g; Fiber: 2g; Protein: 1g; Sodium: 31mg

VEGGIE PÂTÉ

MAKES 3 CUPS PREP TIME: 10 MINUTES COOK TIME: 15 TO 20 MINUTES

CORN FREE
DAIRY FREE
EGG FREE
GLUTEN FREE
NIGHTSHADE FREE
NUT FREE
SOY FREE
PALEO
VEGAN

This highly anti-inflammatory dip makes a lovely alternative to hummus, salsa, or guacamole. Dip crackers and crudités (yes, you'll be dipping your veggies *into* veggies, doubling their nutritional punch), or use as a sandwich spread instead of mustard or mayo.

2 carrots, cut into ½-inch pieces

1 large sweet potato, cut into ½-inch pieces

1 zucchini, cut into ½-inch pieces

1 onion, minced

2 garlic cloves, minced

2 tablespoons water

¾ teaspoon salt

1 Fill a pot with 2 inches of water and insert a steamer basket. Bring the water to a boil over high heat.

2 Add the carrots, sweet potato, and zucchini. Cover and steam for about 10 minutes, or until soft.

3 Meanwhile, in a medium skillet over medium heat, sauté the onion and garlic in the water for about 5 minutes, or until soft.

4 Allow all of the vegetables to cool once cooked.

5 In a food processor, combine the cooked carrots, sweet potato, zucchini, onion, and garlic. Add the salt. Blend until smooth.

6 Refrigerate for at least 1 hour before serving.

COOKING TIP: *When cooking vegetables, cut them into equal sizes. That way, everything cooks at the same time.*

PER SERVING (¼ cup) Calories: 25; Total Fat: 0g; Total Carbohydrates: 6g; Sugar: 2g; Fiber: 1g; Protein: 1g; Sodium:162mg

LEMON-DILL SOUR CREAM

MAKES 1 CUP   PREP TIME: 10 MINUTES   COOK TIME: 0 MINUTES

CORN FREE
DAIRY FREE
EGG FREE
GLUTEN FREE
NIGHTSHADE FREE
SOY FREE
PALEO
VEGAN

Cashews can be whipped into a multitude of tasty dairy-free substitutes—cashew milk, cashew yogurt, cashew cheese, and cashew cream, which is perhaps my favorite cashew variation. You can create a variety of cashew cream flavors, depending on the herbs, spices, and seasoning you decide to use. This recipe is perfect for dolloping on chili or tacos, works great as a dip or sauce for steamed vegetables, and is lovely when spread on gluten-free toast. Cashew cream thickens considerably the longer it sits in the refrigerator, so I like to make a batch the day before serving.

¾ cup cashews, soaked in water for at least 4 hours

¼ cup water

Juice of 1 lemon

Zest of 1 lemon

2 tablespoons chopped fresh dill

¼ teaspoon salt, plus additional as needed

1   Drain the cashews in a mesh sieve and rinse well.

2   In a blender, combine the cashews, water, lemon juice, and lemon zest. Blend until smooth and creamy.

3   Add the dill and salt. Blend again.

4   Taste, and adjust the seasoning if necessary.

5   Refrigerate for at least 1 hour. The cream will thicken in the refrigerator.

SUBSTITUTION TIP: *For those with nut allergies, substitute soaked sunflower seeds.*

PER SERVING (1 tablespoon) Calories: 38; Total Fat: 3g; Total Carbohydrates: 2g; Sugar: 0g; Fiber: 0g; Protein: 1g; Sodium: 37mg

CREAMY LENTIL DIP

MAKES 3 CUPS   PREP TIME: 10 MINUTES   COOK TIME: 15 MINUTES

CORN FREE
DAIRY FREE
EGG FREE
GLUTEN FREE
NIGHTSHADE FREE
NUT FREE
SOY FREE
VEGAN

Chickpeas are a natural for making dips, but they can be difficult for some people to digest. Enter the lentil—a nice alternative to achieve a hummus-like spread without chickpeas. Lentils cook quickly and are filled with protein and fiber, which means they'll fill you up, too. Pair this dip with vegetables or crackers, or spread it on gluten-free toast and top with cucumber slices.

1 cup dried green or brown lentils, rinsed, or 1 (14-ounce) can

2½ cups water, divided

⅓ cup tahini

1 garlic clove

½ teaspoon salt, plus additional as needed

1   In a medium pot, combine the dried lentils with 2 cups of water.

2   Bring to a boil over high heat. Reduce the heat to low and cook for 15 minutes, or until the lentils are tender. If there is water remaining in the pot, drain the lentils.

3   In a food processor, combine the lentils, the remaining ½ cup of water, tahini, garlic, and salt. Blend until smooth and creamy.

4   Taste, and adjust the seasoning if necessary.

SERVING TIP: *Lentils are so delicious and so healthy, but they aren't the most appetizing color. This dip has a greenish, brownish, or greyish hue depending on the type of lentil used. If serving this to a crowd, spruce things up by garnishing with finely chopped parsley, rosemary, basil, or dill.*

PER SERVING (¼ cup) Calories: 101; Total Fat: 4g; Total Carbohydrates: 11g; Sugar: 0g; Fiber: 6g; Protein: 5g; Sodium: 107mg

STRAWBERRY-CHIA JAM

MAKES 1 CUP   PREP TIME: 10 MINUTES   COOK TIME: 8 TO 10 MINUTES

CORN FREE
DAIRY FREE
EGG FREE
GLUTEN FREE
NIGHTSHADE FREE
NUT FREE
SOY FREE
PALEO
VEGAN

Purchased jams are typically doused in white sugar, and often contain added preservatives to thicken them. Both ingredients are unnecessary; fruit, on its own, is both sweet and contains pectin, a natural thickener. Here, I use a moderate amount of maple syrup to enhance the sweetness of the strawberries. If you're new to cooking with chia seeds, note that they swell tremendously in liquid. When dispersed among the strawberry seeds, you won't even notice them.

3 cups fresh strawberries, hulled and halved

¼ cup maple syrup, or raw honey

3 tablespoons chia seeds

1   In a large pot set over medium-low heat, cook the strawberries for 8 to 10 minutes, mashing them lightly with a fork. If the pan gets dry, add 1 or 2 tablespoons of water. Transfer to a blender.

2   Add the maple syrup. Blend until smooth. Pour the mixture into a medium bowl.

3   Stir in the chia seeds.

4   Transfer the jam to a jar. Cover and refrigerate. The jam will thicken as it cools.

SUBSTITUTION TIP: *Any type of berry or stone fruit works in this recipe. Experiment with different kinds of single-fruit jams or mix a variety together.*

PER SERVING (1 tablespoon) Calories: 30; Total Fat: 1g; Total Carbohydrates: 7g; Sugar: 6g; Fiber: 1g; Protein: 1g; Sodium: 0mg

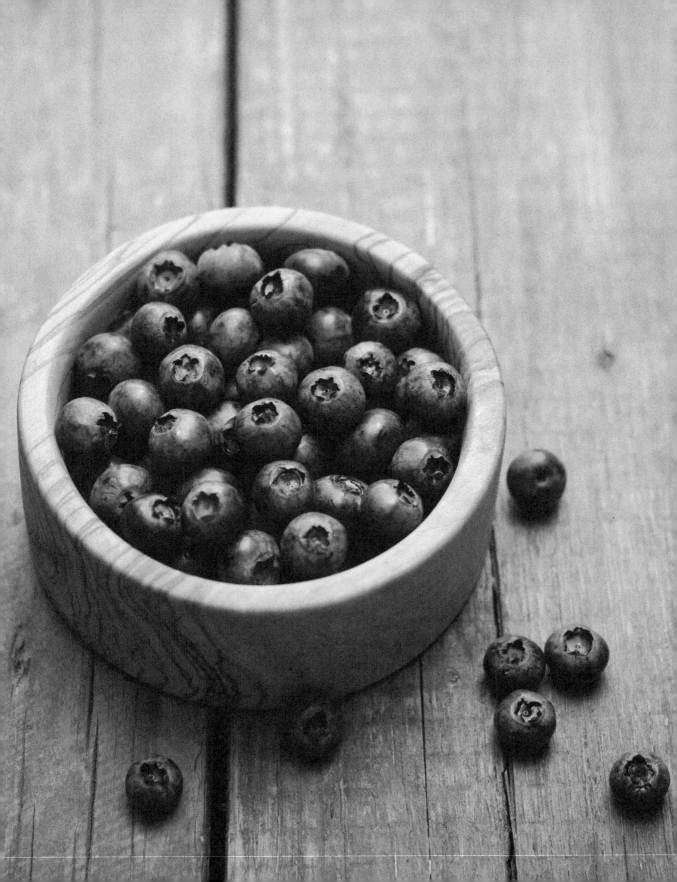

CONVERSION TABLES

VOLUME EQUIVALENTS (LIQUID)

US Standard	US Standard (ounces)	Metric (approximate)
2 tablespoons	1 fl. oz.	30 mL
¼ cup	2 fl. oz.	60 mL
½ cup	4 fl. oz.	120 mL
1 cup	8 fl. oz.	240 mL
1½ cups	12 fl. oz.	355 mL
2 cups or 1 pint	16 fl. oz.	475 mL
4 cups or 1 quart	32 fl. oz.	1 L
1 gallon	128 fl. oz.	4 L

OVEN TEMPERATURES

Fahrenheit (F)	Celsius (C) (approximate)
250°	120°
300°	150°
325°	165°
350°	180°
375°	190°
400°	200°
425°	220°
450°	230°

VOLUME EQUIVALENTS (DRY)

US Standard	Metric (approximate)
⅛ teaspoon	.0.5 mL
¼ teaspoon	1 mL
½ teaspoon	2 mL
¾ teaspoon	4 mL
1 teaspoon	5 mL
1 tablespoon	15 mL
¼ cup	59 mL
⅓ cup	79 mL
½ cup	118 mL
⅔ cup	156 mL
¾ cup	177 mL
1 cup	235 mL
2 cups or 1 pint	475 mL
3 cups	700 mL
4 cups or 1 quart	1 L

WEIGHT EQUIVALENTS

US Standard	Metric (approximate)
½ ounce	15 g
1 ounce	30 g
2 ounces	60 g
4 ounces	115 g
8 ounces	225 g
12 ounces	340 g
16 ounces or 1 pound	455 g

THE DIRTY DOZEN AND THE CLEAN FIFTEEN

A nonprofit watchdog organization called Environmental Working Group (EWG) looks at data supplied by the US Department of Agriculture (USDA) and the Food and Drug Administration (FDA) about pesticide residues. Each year it compiles a list of the best and worst pesticide loads found in commercial crops. You can use these lists to decide which fruits and vegetables to buy organic to minimize your exposure to pesticides and which produce is considered safe enough to buy conventionally. This does not mean they are pesticide-free, though, so wash these fruits and vegetables thoroughly.

These lists change every year, so make sure you look up the most recent one before you fill your shopping cart. You'll find the most recent lists as well as a guide to pesticides in produce at EWG.org/FoodNews.

2015 DIRTY DOZEN

Apples
Celery
Cherry tomatoes
Cucumbers
Grapes
Nectarines
 (imported)
Peaches
Potatoes
Snap peas
 (imported)
Spinach
Strawberries
Sweet bell peppers

In addition to the Dirty Dozen, the EWG added two types of produce contaminated with highly toxic organophosphate insecticides:

Kale/collard greens
Hot peppers

2015 CLEAN FIFTEEN

Asparagus
Avocados
Cabbage
Cantaloupes
 (domestic)
Cauliflower
Eggplants
Grapefruits
Kiwis
Mangoes
Onions
Papayas
Pineapples
Sweet corn
Sweet peas
 (frozen)
Sweet potatoes

RESOURCES

WEBSITES

Dr. Andrew Weil:
www.drweil.com

Dr. Mark Hyman:
www.drhyman.com

Environmental Working Group
Skin-Deep Guide to Cosmetics:
www.ewg.org/skindeep

Environmental Working Group
Guide to Sunscreens:
www.ewg.org/2015sunscreen

Environmental Working Group
Shopper's Guide to Pesticides in
Produce: www.ewg.org/foodnews

Julie Daniluk:
www.juliedaniluk.com

Kris Carr:
www.kriscarr.com

Meghan Telpner:
www.meghantelpner.com

Sondi Bruner Consulting:
www.sondibruner.com

World's Healthiest Foods:
www.whfoods.org

BOOKS

Colbin, Annemarie. *Food and Healing.*
New York: Random House, 1986.

Erasmus, Udo. *Fats that Heal, Fats that Kill.*
Summertown, TN: Alive Books, 1986, 1993.

Murray, Michael and Joseph Pizzorno.
Encyclopedia of Natural Medicine. 2nd ed.
New York: Three Rivers Press, 1998.

Pitchford, Paul. *Healing with Whole Foods.*
3rd ed. Berkeley: North Atlantic Books,
1993, 1996, 2002.

Telpner, Meghan. *UnDiet: Eat Your Way
to Vibrant Health.* Toronto: McClelland &
Stewart, 2013.

Wood, Rebecca. *The New Whole Foods
Encyclopedia.* 2nd ed. New York: Penguin
Group, 2010.

ACKNOWLEDGMENTS

"We have no right to be healed unless we are prepared to return that gift a thousand fold. Health for its own sake is an ego trip. It is a wasted goal; but it gains meaning as a means, an instrument to further the evolution of our consciousness. We must ask ourselves, if we wish to be healthy, what for? To what use will we put our health?"
—Annemarie Colbin, *Food and Healing*

With gratitude to those who remind me of the intention to be of service to others.

REFERENCES

Barański, Marcin, Dominika Średnicka-Tober, Nikolaos Volakakis, Chris Seal, Roy Sanderson, Gavin B. Stewart, Charles Benbrook, et al. "Higher Antioxidant and Lower Cadmium Concentrations and Lower Incidence of Pesticide Residues in Organically Grown Crops: a Systematic Literature Review and Meta-Analyses." *British Journal of Nutrition* 112, no. 5 (September 2014): 794–811.

Benavente-García, O., and J. Castillo. "Update on uses and properties of citrus flavonoids: new findings in anticancer, cardiovascular, and anti-inflammatory activity." *Journal of Agriculture and Food Chemistry* 56, no. 15 (August 13 2008): 6185–205. doi:10.1021/ jf8006568. ePub 2008 July 2.

Colbin, Annemarie. *Food and Healing.* New York: Random House, 1986.

Daniel, Kaayla. "Why Broth is Beautiful: Essential Roles for Proline, Glycine, and Gelatin." The Weston A. Price Foundation. June 18, 2003. Accessed June 29, 2015. www. westonaprice.org/health-topics/ why-broth-is-beautiful-essential-roles-for-proline-glycine-and-gelatin/.

Encyclopedia Britannica. "Inflammation." Last updated April 11, 2014. Accessed June 24, 2015. www. britannica.com/science/inflammation.

Erasmus, Udo. *Fats that Heal, Fats that Kill.* Summertown, TN: Alive Books, 1986, 1993.

Food Allergy Research Education (FARE). "Allergens." Accessed July 8, 2015. www.foodallergy.org/allergens.

Ford, E.S. "Does Exercise Reduce Inflammation? Physical Activity and C-Reactive Protein Among U.S. Adults." *Epidemiology* 13, no. 5 (September 2002): 561–8.

GMO Compass. "USA 2013: No Reversal of Trend—Farmers Stick to Their Varieties of GM Crops." May 21, 2014. Accessed June 27, 2015. www.gmo-compass.org/eng/agri_biotechnology/ gmo_planting/506.usa_cultivation_gm_ plants_2013.html.

Harvard Health Publications: Harvard Medical School. "What You Eat Can Fuel or Cool Inflammation, a Key Driver of Heart Disease, Diabetes, and Other Chronic Conditions." Last updated February 2007. Accessed June 24, 2015. www.health.harvard.edu/ family_health_guide/what-you-eat-can-fuel-or-cool-inflammation-a-key-driver-of-heart-disease-diabetes-and-other-chronic-conditions.

Health Canada. "Food Allergies." Accessed July 8, 2015. www.hc-sc. gc.ca/fn-an/securit/allerg/fa-aa/index-eng.php.

Hyman, Mark. "Inflammation: How to Cool the Fire Inside You That's Making You Fat and Diseased." Dr. Mark Hyman. January 27, 2012. Accessed June 24, 2015. www.drhyman.com/2012/01/27/inflammation-how-to-cool-the-fire-inside-you-thats-making-you-fat-and-diseased/.

Hyman, Mark. "Is Your Body Burning Up With Hidden Inflammation?" The Huffington Post. September 24, 2009. Accessed June 24, 2015. www.huffingtonpost.com/dr-mark-hyman/is-your-body-burning-up-w_b_269717.html.

Institute for Agriculture and Trade Policy. "No Time to Lose: 147 Studies Supporting Public Health Action to Reduce Antibiotic Overuse in Food Animals." October 30, 2012. Accessed June 28, 2015. www.iatp.org/documents/no-time-to-lose-147-studies-supporting-public-health-action-to-reduce-antibiotic-overuse-i.

Jiang, Yu, Sheng-Hui Wu, Xiao-Ou Shu, Yong-Bing Xiang, Bu-Tian Ji, Ginger L. Milne, Qiuyin Cai, et. al. "Cruciferous Vegetable Intake Is Inversely Correlated with Circulating Levels of Proinflammatory Markers in Women." *Journal of the Academy of Nutrition and Dietetics* 114, no. 5 (May 2014): 700–8. Published online 2014 Mar 13. doi:10.1016/j.jand.2013.12.019.

Lipski, Elizabeth. *Digestive Wellness*. 3rd ed. New York: McGraw Hill, 2005.

Mateljan, George. *The World's Healthiest Foods*. Seattle: George Mateljan Foundation, 2007.

Mayo Clinic. "Food Allergies: Understanding Food Labels." February 6, 2014. Accessed July 8, 2015. www.mayoclinic.org/diseases-conditions/food-allergy/in-depth/food-allergies/art-20045949.

Medical News Today. "Inflammation: Causes, Symptoms, and Treatment." Last updated May 25, 2015. Accessed June 24, 2015. www.medicalnewstoday.com/articles/248423.php.

Medical News Today. "What Are the Health Benefits of Rosemary?" Updated September 5, 2014. Accessed July 21, 2015. www.medicalnewstoday.com/articles/266370.php.

Mercola, Joseph. "Bone Broth—One of Your Most Healing Diet Staples." Mercola.com. December 16, 2013. Accessed June 29, 2015. www.articles.mercola.com/sites/articles/archive/2013/12/16/bone-broth-benefits.aspx.

Mercola.com. "Why Grassfed Animal Products Are Better For You." Accessed June 28, 2015. www.mercola.com/beef/health_benefits.htm.

Mitoshi, M., I. Kuriyama, H. Nakayama, H. Miyazato, K. Sugimoto, Y. Kobayashi, T. Jippo, et al. "Suppression of Allergic and Inflammatory Responses by Essential Oils Derived From Herbal Plants and Citrus Fruits." *International Journal of Molecular Medicine* 33, no. 6 (June 2014): 1643–51. doi:10.3892/ijmm.2014.1720. ePub 2014 Mar 31.

Morris, Alanna, Dorothy Coverson, Lucy Fike, Yusuf Ahmed, Neli Stoyanova, W. Craig Hooper, Gary Gibbons, et al. "Sleep Quality and Duration are Associated with Higher Levels of Inflammatory Biomarkers: the META-Health Study." *Circulation* 122, (2010): A17806.

Murakami, A., Y. Nakamura, Y. Ohto, M. Yano, T. Koshiba, K. Koshimizu, H. Tokuda, et al. "Suppressive Effects of Citrus Fruits on Free Radical Generation and Nobiletin, an Anti-inflammatory Polymethoxyflavonoid." *BioFactors* 12, no. 1–4 (2000): 187–92.

Murray, Michael, and Joseph Pizzorno. *Encyclopedia of Natural Medicine.* 2nd ed. New York: Three Rivers Press, 1998.

National Heart, Lung, and Blood Institute. "What Are the Health Risks of Overweight and Obesity?" Last updated July 13, 2012. Accessed July 8, 2015. www.nhlbi.nih.gov/health/health-topics/topics/obe/risks.

Nett, Amy. "How Resistant Starch Will Help to Make You Healthier and Thinner." ChrisKresser.com. August 4, 2014. Accessed July 14, 2015. www.chriskresser.com/how-resistant-starch-will-help-to-make-you-healthier-and-thinner.

Ogawa, Kishiko, Kiyoshi Sanada, Shuichi Machida, Mitsuharu Okutsu, and Katsuhiko Suzuki. "Resistance Exercise Training-Induced Muscle Hypertrophy was Associated with Reduction of Inflammatory Markers in Elderly Women." *Mediators of Inflammation* 2010 (2010): 7 pages. doi:10.1155/2010/171023.

Perlmutter, David. *Grain Brain.* New York: Little, Brown and Company, September 2013.

PubMed Health. "What Is an Inflammation?" Last updated January 2015. Accessed June 24, 2015. www.ncbi.nlm.nih.gov/pubmedhealth/PMH0072482/.

Rakoff-Nahoum, Seth. "Why Cancer and Inflammation?" *Yale Journal of Biology and Medicine* 79, no. 3–4 (2006 December): 123–130.

Rodale's Organic Life. "The 10 Healthiest Food Pairings." April 9, 2012. Accessed July 17, 2015. www.rodalesorganiclife.com/food/food-pairings.

Science Daily. "How Stress Influences Disease: Study Reveals Inflammation As the Culprit." April 12, 2012. Accessed June 24, 2015. http://www.sciencedaily.com/releases/2012/04/120402162546.htm.

Sisson, Mark. "The Relationship Between Exercise and Inflammation (and What It Means for Your Workouts)." Mark's Daily Apple. January 17, 2012. Accessed July 9, 2015. www.marksdailyapple.com/the-relationship-between-exercise-and-inflammation-and-what-it-means-for-your-workouts/#axzz3fQhfvnkJ.

Trafton, Anne. "Study Details a Link Between Inflammation and Cancer." MIT News. January 15, 2015. Accessed July 8, 2015. www.newsoffice.mit.edu/2015/link-between-inflammation-and-cancer-0115.

Tsai, Jo-Ting, Liu Hui-Ching, and Yue-Hwa Chen. "Suppression of Inflammatory Mediators by Cruciferous Vegetable-Derived Indole-3-Carbinol and Phenylethyl Isothiocyanate in Lipopolysaccharide-Activated Macrophages." Mediators of Inflammation (2010): 293642. doi:10.1155/2010/293642.

University of Maryland Medical Center. "Omega-3 Fatty Acids." June 24, 2013. Accessed June 24, 2015. www.umm.edu/health/medical/altmed/supplement/omega3-fatty-acids.

Wilson, James. *Adrenal Fatigue: The 21st Century Syndrome.* Petaluma, CA: Smart Publications, 2001.

Wood, Rebecca. *The New Whole Foods Encyclopedia.* 2nd ed. New York: Penguin Group, 2010.

World's Healthiest Foods. "Eating Healthy With Cruciferous Vegetables." Accessed July 8, 2015. www.whfoods.com/genpage.php?tname=btnews&dbid=126.

RECIPE INDEX

INDEX

ABOUT THE AUTHOR

SONDI BRUNER is a holistic nutritionist, writer, food blogger, and recipe developer who specializes in digestive issues and allergen-friendly diets. She lives in Vancouver, British Columbia, with her husband and fur baby.